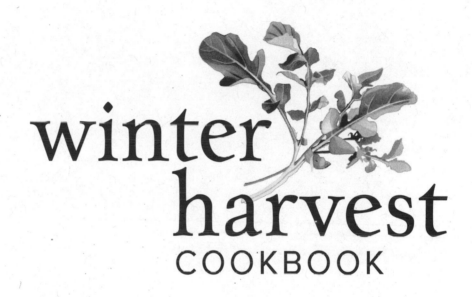

winter
harvest
COOKBOOK

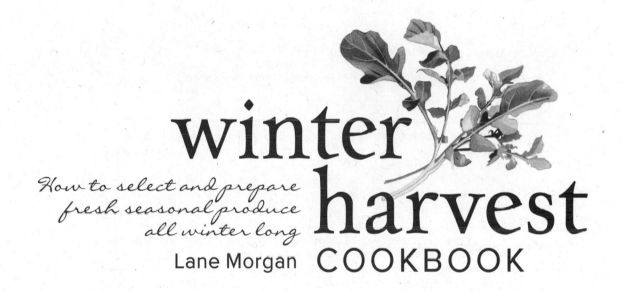

winter harvest

*How to select and prepare
fresh seasonal produce
all winter long*

Lane Morgan

COOKBOOK

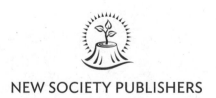

NEW SOCIETY PUBLISHERS

Inquiries regarding requests to reprint all or part of *Winter Harvest Cookbook* should be addressed to New Society Publishers at the address below.

To order directly from the publishers, please call toll-free (North America) 1-800-567-6772, or order online at www.newsociety.com

Any other inquiries can be directed by mail to:
New Society Publishers
P.O. Box 189, Gabriola Island, BC V0R 1X0, Canada
(250) 247-9737

New Society Publishers' mission is to publish books that contribute in fundamental ways to building an ecologically sustainable and just society, and to do so with the least possible impact on the environment, in a manner that models this vision. We are committed to doing this not just through education, but through action. Our printed, bound books are printed on Forest Stewardship Council-certified acid-free paper that is **100% post-consumer recycled** (100% old growth forest-free), processed chlorine free, and printed with vegetable-based, low-VOC inks, with covers produced using FSC-certified stock. New Society also works to reduce its carbon footprint, and purchases carbon offsets based on an annual audit to ensure a carbon neutral footprint. For further information, or to browse our full list of books and purchase securely, visit our website at: www.newsociety.com

LIBRARY AND ARCHIVES CANADA CATALOGUING IN PUBLICATION

Morgan, Lane, 1949–
Winter harvest cookbook : how to select and prepare fresh seasonal produce all winter long / Lane Morgan. — Rev. and updated 20th anniversary ed.

Includes bibliographical references and indexes.
ISBN 978-0-86571-679-7   eISBN: 978-1-55092-458-9

1. Cooking (Vegetables).   I. Title.

TX801.M68 2010   641.6'5   C2010-904787-7

NEW SOCIETY PUBLISHERS
www.newsociety.com

Mixed Sources
Product group from well-managed forests, controlled sources and recycled wood or fiber
www.fsc.org Cert no. SW-COC-000952
© 1996 Forest Stewardship Council
FSC

To my daughters,
Laurel and Deshanna

contents

acknowledgments

A lifetime of cooking and gardening with friends and family could make this list as long as the book itself, but there are some people I particularly want to thank. Carolyn Dale and Tim Pilgrim, for kiwis, rhubarb, and great meals; Mary Jean Wiegert and Bruce Underwood for rutabagas and a memorable evening in their fabulous kitchen; Robert (Goldtooth) Ray, for taste testing both the successes and the stranger experiments; Mark Musick, Bruce Naftaly, Jon Kemnitzer, Deb Anderson-Frey, Marilyn Lewis, Gale Lawrence, Bill Bowes, and Kristen Barber for recipes and encouragement, Curt Madison, for 40+ years of friendship and that moose roast; Bruce Brown, for Sumas days and for reminding me about my garden journals; my friend and agent Anne Depue; and my family—Deshanna Brown, Laurel, Ronny and Hailey Tull, and Andrew Tull—for loving me.

preface to
the new edition

When I wrote the first *Winter Harvest*, I was married with young children. We lived on a homestead farm on the Canadian border where we milked the cow, made our own butter, raised calves, chickens, turkeys and hogs and grew nearly all our own vegetables and fruit. I cooked on a woodstove and had yet to use a food processor or a microwave.

I've regretted that I didn't keep a consistent journal of that time, but when I reread the book, I realized that it does serve as a kind of record. It has lots of slow-cooked recipes of the sort that can simmer for hours at the back of the woodstove. Its meat dishes featured beef, chicken, and pork, which we raised, rather than seafood, which we didn't. I don't eat lamb or veal, so there are no recipes for them in either edition. Most recipes are simple and flexible. I was a homesteader, a writer and editor, a part-time professor, and a wife and mom. I didn't have the time or the audience for elaborate dishes. But they also reflect my lifelong interest in world cuisines. (This was first manifest when I was four, living in Mexico, and entranced with fire-roasted grasshoppers, and it has only increased with time.)

Twenty years later, I am single and a grandmother. I teach high school, and I live on a small lot in town. I still garden year-round, but the livestock is gone along with the woodstove. I have a microwave, a food processor, and even a bread machine. What hasn't changed is my appreciation of local food and sustainable practices, and my conviction that eating with the seasons is best for our health, our palate and our planet. I'm writing this in April. The local stores and even my food co-op are stocked with California strawberries and Mexican tomatoes, both big and beautiful and nearly interchangeable in their lack of flavor. My garden kale, on the other hand, is making its last, sweetest growth spurt before it goes to seed. It's much tastier than those far-from-home tomatoes, and it doesn't cost $3.50 a pound. At the farmers market on Saturdays, I can already get collards, leeks, beets, spinach, potatoes, radishes and salad mixes, plus local bread, cheese, eggs, meat and fish. The growth of the Bellingham Farmers Market, from the 1980s when I used to sell my extra leeks and chard from a makeshift booth next to the bus station to its current iconic status as the place to meet, greet, and eat on Saturdays from April through December, has fueled a corresponding explosion of small farms and market gardens. "Big A" agriculture is under siege in Northwest Washington as elsewhere, with acreage dwindling under pressure from development, but the number of small truck farms and Community Supported Agriculture programs is growing yearly.

Town dwellers are also in on the act. Although I no longer raise chickens, on my city block alone there are laying flocks, domestic ducks, and miniature Nigerian milk goats. Mine is far from the only front yard where edibles including strawberries, rainbow chard, red orach, and blueberry bushes are thriving among the more traditional ornamentals. I have potatoes growing in a tub on my deck, apple trees espaliered along the fence, hardy kiwis twining with the clematis and climbing up into the overgrown California lilac. Artichokes spike up next to foxgloves, and raspberries arch over the tulips and daylilies, all watered from my collection of rain barrels. Our neighborhood coffee stand got so many requests for their grounds that they now bag up their little discs of spent espresso grounds and leave them out by the alley for gardeners to pick up. Lacking manure, I use the high-nitrogen grounds to jumpstart my compost, which is slowly converting the long-neglected dirt in my yard into actual soil.

In the first edition, I wrote about environmental and nutritional reasons to eat locally produced food. Since then the alarms of global climate change have added urgency to this idea. I don't feel competent to argue the finer points. I recently had a delicious collard wrap at a local vegan/raw food restaurant. Did the avocado and pumpkin seeds in the filling (both shipped in from elsewhere) ultimately have a lower carbon footprint than an egg from my neighbor's hen? Was the agave syrup for my tea better for the planet than local honey, or even than refined sugar made from Washington-grown beets? I just don't know. I do know, however, that flying fresh corn in from Florida in March, as my neighborhood grocer did last year, is just plain crazy. Someone else would have to calculate the environmental cost per kernel for a dish where most of the shipped weight goes right into the trash. Or the hourly diminishing likelihood that it would actually taste anything like real corn. But for certain, half the magic of fresh sweet corn is the waiting.

When I had room to grow it myself, the corn vigil began with the seed catalogs in January, when we decided between Burgundy Delight and Silver Queen. Then we had to wait until our heavy soil was dry enough to work. Some years we could start early enough to fulfill the local mantra for a good harvest: "knee-high by the Fourth of July." By early August, the drama centered around outwitting the raccoons, whose idea of "harvest ready" preceded ours, and who could trash a small corn patch in an evening. Finally the day came when the ears felt heavy, the kernels were plump and tight. It was time to boil water in the biggest pot we had. Really fresh corn is wonderful raw, but if you at least heat it through, the homemade butter and pesto melt into the ears. We gorged on corn for weeks. We steamed it, roasted it, and scraped it off the cobs for fritters and chowder. The hogs chomped the cobs, and the cows drooled copiously over the stalks. Our daughters chewed on the stalks, too; they taste like corn syrup flavored with grass. When the late September corn patch was down to some overripe monster ears and a few skinny semi-pollinated late bloomers, it was time to move on to apples and Brussels sprouts, and to dream about next year's corn.

There are no corn recipes in this book, no fresh tomatoes or sweet peppers, no green beans or eggplant, no strawberries or sugar snap peas. But implicit in the celebration of one season is the anticipation of the next. It's like a secret spice that adds flavor to what we have right now. "Hunger in a garden has a way of relating to the garden," wrote Angelo Pellegrini. These recipes are written for that hunger, the kind that comes from the food we have before us.

introduction to the 1990 edition

This book got its start more than 10 years ago, when I first encountered Binda Colebrook's *Winter Gardening* in the Maritime Northwest. I liked the idea of extending my gardening season, and I began some tentative experiments in my backyard in Seattle. When we moved to the country in 1979, I learned to my delight that Binda lived and farmed nearby. We became friends, and I helped with research for the second editing of *Winter Gardening*.

Under her tutelage my winter garden flourished, but then I had a new problem. What was I supposed to do with all that chard and kale and salsify? Customers at the Bellingham Farmers Market, where I sold my surplus, had the same trouble. A lumpy Jerusalem artichoke, however sweet and crisp, somehow doesn't inspire the kind of culinary confidence that comes from a perfect, vine-ripe tomato. But on the other hand, a perfect Jerusalem artichoke is available and affordable in Bellingham in December, while a good tomato is not.

I began to hunt up recipes for my new crops and to invent a few of my own. The process was very satisfying. For one thing, I have more patience for cooking in winter. Since I can't garden in the dark, I might as well be inside. For another, food seems more important then. We want to gather our friends at the table and keep the gloom away. I feel victorious when I come back from the muddy garden, clutching a bunch of leeks and chard, ready for adventure.

Why winter vegetables

Everything is best in its season. Whether your produce is from your garden or from the market, the best value for your money, your palate, and your health is in the crops that flourish most naturally. In summer, this is easy advice to follow. Who wouldn't choose fresh raspberries over stored apples in July? In winter, what used to be an inescapable cycle of seasonal food has begun to seem an exercise in self-discipline. It's hard not to be seduced by the ever-increasing array of foodstuffs from someone else's summer. But locally grown Brussels sprouts, properly cooked, really will taste better than corn trucked in from Florida.

Furthermore, the more local our food, the better we can assess its real costs and benefits. For example, nearly half the tomatoes sold in the United States between December and May come from the Culiacán Valley in Mexico. Americans want their produce spotless—especially when they are paying top dollar—so the tomatoes (and the workers who harvest them) are repeatedly and heavily sprayed with pesticides and fungicides. Then the tomatoes are picked green, bathed in chlorine, gassed with ethylene to stimulate reddening (but not ripening), and shipped across the continent, losing vitamins every step of the way.

When these tomatoes end up on the shelf in Seattle, they are still legally fresh, but they are neither tasty nor nutritious, and they may not even be safe. Assuming that they actually have been tested for violations of pesticide regulations—and that's not a safe assumption—they will have gone into the salad long before the lab reports are in. If the price tag on those tomatoes included the real costs in health and environmental damage, the product would be a lot less alluring. (Long-distance organic produce, though preferable, is not likely to rate much better nutritionally.)

Fortunately, there is no need to put purity before pleasure at the dinner table. When it comes to winter produce, good sense and good taste can go together.

What winter vegetables

The vegetables featured in this book reach their peak of flavor in cool weather. Corn, tomatoes, eggplant, green beans, peppers, and zucchini are all fruits and seeds, the crown of the plant's creation. It takes a lot of energy to produce them, and that energy comes from long, sunny days. When the nights are long and the days are cool, most plants forgo flowers and stick with the basics: leaves and roots. Spinach, lettuce, cauliflower, mustard in its infinite varieties, kale and collards, and leeks all reach culinary perfection before they flower. If their development is hurried along by too much light and heat, their vitality will suffer along with their flavor.

Beets, carrots, parsnips, salsify, scorzonera, celeriac, and others are biennials. Their roots store the nutrients that will get the dormant plants through the winter. In many cases, cold weather improves the taste, converting some of the starches in the roots to sugar. If they don't end up on your table first, the plants will draw from these high-energy reserves come spring to produce flowers and seeds.

Crops such as winter squash, potatoes, and sweet potatoes mostly ripen in summer, but unlike tomatoes or green beans, they actually are improved in many cases by some time in storage.

This book is dedicated to the pleasures of fresh food in the winter season. But I admit that even in the Pacific Northwest, which is a mecca for cool weather crops, total fidelity to a fresh seasonal table would be pretty restrictive. After all, cardboard tomatoes sell not because anybody really likes them, but because people crave an alternative to rutabagas. I'm not willing to do without lemons and oranges, winter or summer, and many of my favorite recipes call for canned tomatoes. Though fashion may scorn it, canned and frozen produce is often a better choice than globetrotting "fresh." A tomato that was picked ripe and canned will be just as tasty cooked as one that was picked green and shipped, at a fraction of the price. (The vitamin C will be long gone in either case.) Likewise, fresh spinach is no nutritional powerhouse unless it's locally grown and you plan to eat it within a day or two. Otherwise, buy frozen and save yourself the cleaning time. Or skip spinach until you can find some worth eating.

All cooking was seasonal until recent times, so winter vegetables are central to many classic recipes. French *garbure*, Italian *bagna cauda*, Brazilian *feijoada*, Japanese *tsukemono*—all are based on cold-weather stalwarts like cabbage, cardoons, collards, and turnips. A vegetable like kale reveals an amazing number of uses and attributes as it moves from the "brose" soups of Scotland to the *caldo verde* of Portugal to the stews of Central Africa, and across the ocean to Southern soul food. Other standard winter staples—including potatoes, yams, and rutabagas—have a much greater culinary range than most of us know.

The many gardeners who have been inspired by *Winter Gardening* and other guides have been active in reviving old recipes and inventing new ones. As every gardener knows, a bumper crop can be a potent source of inspiration.

I have tried to keep esoteric ingredients and complicated procedures to a minimum. If you garden, you have already done plenty of work before the food hits the table, and if you live in a rural area, you can't just run down to the corner if a recipe calls for a dash of Pernod. On the other hand, I love trying new tastes. Moroccan pickled lemons won't be easy to find at the supermarket, but they are simple and cheap to prepare at home.

Where to get them

The more familiar winter vegetables can be found in any supermarket. Whenever possible, buy produce that is locally grown. You will get fresher, higher-quality products, and you will be investing in the future of agriculture in your region. As a local buyer, you also have more power. Complaints and suggestions from consumers reach the local farmer in a hurry.

Keep in mind that local does not mean dirt cheap. Growing crops for winter and spring harvest takes skill. Harvesting them is cold, wet, dirty work. Farmers aren't going to do it if it doesn't pay. Unlike large-scale meat and grain—the true production costs of which are obscured by irrigation subsidies and other political hat tricks—locally produced vegetables have to pay their own way. Eating in season is still economical, but don't expect giveaway prices.

Specialty grocers and farmers markets are good sources of lesser-known or highly perishable foods. Some small-scale growers will produce on contract: you commit yourself at planting time to a certain number of celeriacs and pick them up in the fall.

If you are a gardener, consider extending your season. Proper attention to vegetable varieties and planting times can give your salads in November and leeks in March. Gardeners in many regions can harvest vegetables every day of the year, and cold frames and greenhouses make winter crops possible even in severe climates. Apartment dwellers can keep themselves in salads and herbs with some pots in a sunny window.

I live just south of the Canadian border in Sumas, Washington, where the murky winter weather common to the Maritime Northwest is enlivened every year or two with screaming winds and zero-degree blizzards that can swallow cars and (one memorable year) snowplows. A more typical January day might have eight hours of feeble daylight and a high temperature of 25°F. Nevertheless, between November and April, my garden has produced broccoli, Brussels sprouts, kale, collards, various cabbages, leeks, green onions, leaf celery, Swiss chard, lettuce, endive, spinach, sorrel, cauliflower, Jerusalem artichokes, cardoons, celeriac, parsnips, salsify, and more. Other late crops, such as potatoes, carrots, and winter squash, are stored inside, away from pest and frosts. I certainly don't raise all those vegetables every year, but I can nearly always count on something.

Because winter plants are hardy, it isn't surprising that many of them flourish on their own. Burdock, chicory, nettles, fennel, and dandelions are all welcome additions to winter or early spring meal, and I have seen them growing in vacant lots in Seattle as well as in the countryside.

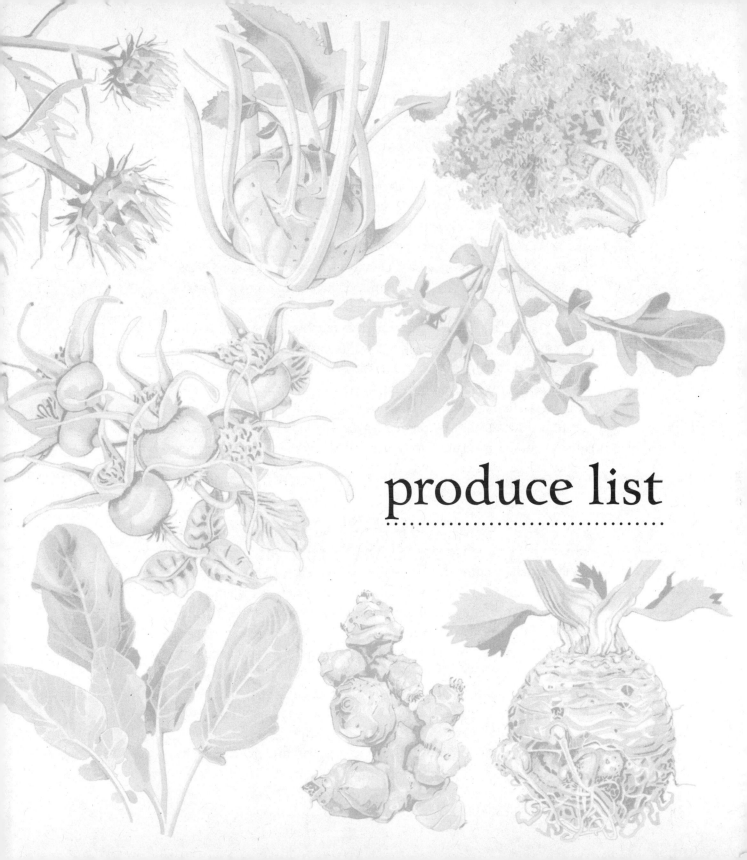

produce list

amaranth

(een choi, bledo, alegria)

AMARANTHUS SPP.

. . . .

As amaranth, this fleshy green or reddish potherb has been enjoying a modest renaissance, particularly for the nutritional virtues of its tiny seeds. As pigweed, amaranth is still the same old garden weed it ever was. It is up early in the spring, and the young leaves are a reasonable substitute for spinach. As they get tougher and stronger tasting, leaves should be treated like chard. I add the odd bit of amaranth to stir-fries and mixed-green dishes such as hortopita.

Most country dwellers probably have some pigweed around for the foraging, so you can check out the flavor before committing yourself to a garden crop. Commercial seed yields a variety of colors and sizes, making amaranth a popular choice for edible landscapers. An ornamental variety, often sold in flower catalogs as a giant Love Lies Bleeding, has red leaves that look lovely in a spring salad. Another, marketed by Territorial Seeds as Double Color, has purple leaves with green edges.

apples

. . . .

Apples are a late-summer to late-fall crop by nature. Cold storage and wax coverings (and shipping from New Zealand) make them available year-round. The trick for gardeners and local eaters is to find out what grows best, and keeps best, in your region without commercial technology. Some varieties, such as Melrose, will keep improving in flavor until Christmas and keep in your refrigerator until March or April. Other late ripeners and good keepers include Ashmead's Kernal, Fuji, and Idareds, which sometimes last until May.

Conventionally grown apples regularly appear on the Dirty Dozen lists for pesticide and herbicide residues, and even here in

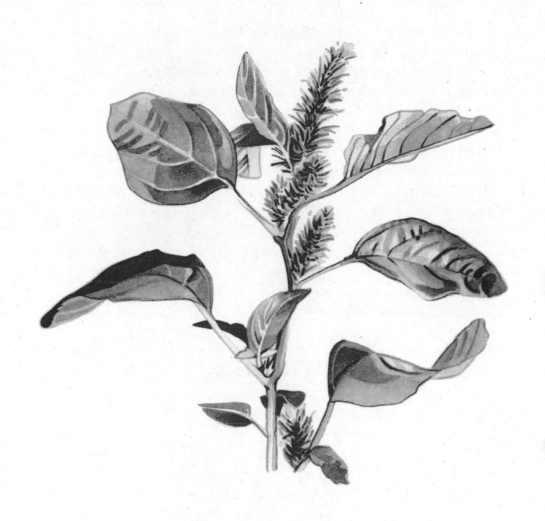

amaranth
·······························

Washington state, which produces more than 100 million boxes of commercial apples per year, quality apples aren't cheap. So it pays to grow your own if you can. I have three mini-dwarf trees espaliered to my deck railing, the only way I could figure to fit them into my small, mostly shady yard. My neighbors up the block have a columnar apple tree in a pot on each side of their gate. Back on the farm, we had more apples than we could handle. We made gallons of cider and sauce and barely made a dent. I still remember the horrified response I got on a trip to Cuba when I told our translator that we fed windfall apples to our cows. An apple there was a precious and rare treat. On the other hand, they had so many luscious papaya that they invented recipes for green ones just to keep from getting bored. When I pine for fresh peaches in winter, but I have apples instead, I try to keep that in mind. One person's excess is another one's treasure.

arugula
(garden rocket, misticanza)
Eruca sativa

Documentation of arugula in the kitchen goes back to at least the late medieval period. After a period of intense trendiness in the 1980s, it seems to have settled into a modest popularity as a salad green. I love the sesame-pepper taste of the young plants, especially when mixed with the blander corn salad that grows nearby in my winter garden. Mature plants are too hot to eat with pleasure, but if you leave a few for seed, you'll have arugula all spring and fall.

Like many of their leafy ilk, arugulas interbreed with enthusiasm, and the flavor gets erratic after a few years. Then it's time to reseed from commercial stock and start again.

When buying arugula, look for bright green, young plants; wash them gently and thoroughly and use right away. Dry the leaves carefully; they can't take rough handling.

beets

BETA VULGARIS

Spring is the time for succulent little baby beets, steamed, with maybe a dab of butter. In the fall, you want types that hold their sugar content well and do not develop a woody core. Gardeners can experiment with mangel-wurzel and other sugar-beet types, which are huge, hardy, and very sweet. Before corn syrup gained hegemony over the world of domestic sweeteners, sugar beets were a major farm crop in Eastern Washington and Idaho. Golden beets, such as Touchstone Gold, lack the slightly metallic tang that puts some people off the red ones and are beautiful in their own right. I think they are a better choice for roasting, as they seem more apt to caramelize deliciously as they cook, but I haven't subjected this perception to a scientific test. There are also white beets, which I have not tried. West Coast Seeds in Delta, B.C., has an especially good beet selection. (See Resources.)

brussels sprouts

BRASSICA OLERACEA VAR. GEMIFERA

Brussels sprouts are at their best in winter, as frost sweetens them. Hardy European varieties can stand bitter weather; I have broken through frozen snow to harvest them and seen them survive the thaw to produce some more. Whether buying or harvesting, look for tight, green buttons of medium size, and once you have them in your kitchen, do not overcook. Most Brussels-sprout haters got that way from an encounter with the pale, rank-tasting victims of too much boiling. Try roasting, steaming or sautéing instead.

If you grow your own, don't spurn the elongating heads as the plants go to flower in the spring. They have a slightly peppery taste and are delicious in stir-fries or quickly steamed and drizzled with butter and lemon.

cabbage

BRASSICA SPP.

. . . .

Cabbages take a bewildering variety of forms, and they are cool-weather crops par excellence. Herewith an informal grouping:

Asian types

Large, crisp, mild-tasting Chinese or Napa cabbage (*Brassica pekinensis* var. *cylindrica*) is sort of the iceberg lettuce of the cabbage family. It shares another characteristic in that it is tricky to grow, and I have given up trying. Fortunately, it is widely available. Individual heads can be huge, but it keeps fairly well under refrigeration, so don't hesitate. Any excess can be made into *kim chee*.

Bok choy and its cousins, with pale, thick stalks and dark green leaves, have a bit more flavor and are easier to grow because they do not need to form a head. Seed catalogs and Asian markets will introduce you to an ever-growing array of other types, shading by flavor into the mustards, which I have arbitrarily gathered into a separate section (see mustards). In general, the larger and paler the produce, the milder the taste, so you might tailor your experiments accordingly.

European types

Savoy cabbages, exceptionally hardy and very beautiful, are one of the best arguments for a winter garden. They are not often seen in supermarkets in the US, since their long growing season and relatively short shelf life make them problematic for agribusiness, but they are troupers in the garden. The crinkled ("savoyed") leaves evidently provide some cold protection (savoyed spinach is also a winter variety). The flavor is milder and the leaves less fibrous than those of ordinary cabbage. Not recommended for a mayonnaise-laden coleslaw, but otherwise you can try it in most recipes calling for cabbage. It is especially nice for stuffed cabbage because the softer leaves are easier to handle without breaking.

A cross-section of red cabbage is so lovely, it's worth getting one just for that. Its beauty is a factor when used fresh in salads. Red cabbages tend to be a bit firmer and harder than their green counterparts and may require longer cooking if tenderness is the issue.

Green cabbage should have hard, firm heads, medium-sized rather than huge. A big one might be dominated by a huge core, and you won't know until you've cut it open. Gardeners have the option of fast-maturing, loose-headed spring cabbage, but these varieties seldom make it to market.

Space and fertile soil are two priorities if you want to grow your own cabbage. They like lots of nutrients, and in turn, pests love them. Cabbage root-fly maggot was the biggest challenge when I still had room for a cabbage patch, but aphids and caterpillars got their licks in too. All of these pests can be managed organically, but it takes some skill and discipline, at least in the Maritime Northwest.

cardoons

(cardone, cardon)

CYNARA CARDUNCULUS

Food historian Waverly Root says that European women in the Middle Ages ate cardoons to ensure the birth of a boy. I eat them for the mild artichoke taste, provided in bulk by the burly stalks. Cardoons are a giant form of thistle, related to artichokes but hardier and—because one eats the stems rather then the flower buds—more prolific. A happy cardoon plant can top six feet and is likely to outlive its artichoke cousin, lasting close to a decade.

Cardoons are most common in Northern Italian cooking, and have immigrated along with Italians to Argentina, where they are also widely served. They are used in bagna cauda, smorfati, and other traditional dishes. European growers have more varieties to choose from, and may concentrate spineless forms, or on subtleties of flavor. Angelo Pellegrini, the revered Seattle English professor, writer and gardener, raised cardoons successfully for many years, and he made an eloquent case for them in his fine book, *The Food Lover's Garden*. Pellegrini also cooked with the ubiquitous Canadian thistle, known by more forgiving souls than me as "wild cardoons." I haven't tried this and probably won't, given their nasty spines.

Cardoon stalks will keep a week refrigerated in a plastic bag. Strip and trim the stalks before cooking. The central ones are the mildest.

carrots
DAUCA CAROTA

If you garden, you can indulge in the great range of carrot sizes, colors, and flavors, and plan your menus according to type. Most kinds are winter hardy, and Nantes types have a particularly good reputation as a winter keeper. My Purple Haze plantings—day-glo violet on the outside and orange within—made it through a 14°F freeze last winter and were crisp and sweet in the spring.

cauliflower
BRASSICA OLERACEA BOTRYTIS

Home gardeners have a tremendous range of cauliflowers to choose from. If you are determined, you can harvest them almost continuously from September to April. The determination comes in because they can be tricky to grow. They like rich soil, lots of water, and coolish temperatures. Summer in Ketchikan is just about ideal. Further south, overwintered varieties are sown just when the cabbage root-fly maggot and cabbage worms are hitting their peak, adding challenges especially for organic growers.

Shoppers should look for the obvious: firm heads that have not begun to separate or discolor. I can't tell any consistent difference in taste between the modest heads and the gargantuan ones, so let menu-planning convenience be your guide and buy what you can use right away. Freshness is what matters. I did a roasted cauliflower taste test using one picked that morning and another (also organic and locally grown) that had spent a few days in the crisper drawer. The results were dramatic, the difference between good and wonderful.

Specialty cauliflowers—green, golden or purple—are now available in groceries and farmers markets as well as seed catalogs. You can take advantage of these plant breeder's fantasies in an eye-catching antipasto plate. The purple ones turn green when cooked.

celeriac

(celery root, célery-rave)

A PIUM GRAVEOLENS VAR. RAPACEUM

A member of the parsley family (as is celery), celeriac is grown for its bulbous root. It has a mild flavor, rather like the blanched heart of a regular celery. I wish it well as a supermarket vegetable, since it is slow to grow and hard to clean, two drawbacks for the home gardener. It keeps well, though, and the size is more convenient than those massive store-bought celery bunches that inevitably grow limp in the back of my refrigerator.

Small, gnarly roots are good for soups and stews. If you grow or buy nice big ones, you can try the many Continental recipes for purées and rémoulades.

celery

APIUM GRAVEOLENS

Leaf celery, available from Reimers Seeds and a few other specialty catalogs, is surprisingly hardy and much easier to grow than regular celery. With a little mulching, it will survive all but the fiercest Northwest winters and produce new growth in early spring. The flavor is much stronger than that of commercial celery. Too much can overpower your pot roast, and munching it raw is out of the question. Cut the amount in half if you are using it in place of regular celery.

chestnuts

CASTENEA SPP.

North American chestnut production is making a modest comeback after the blight that devastated American trees in the early twentieth century. Despite their rich, mealy taste, chestnuts are much lower in fat than any other commercial nut. This is good news both for nutrition and versatility, as dried chestnuts can be ground into a baking flour that is much more versatile than oilier ground nut mixtures. Also unlike other nuts, chestnuts are rarely eaten raw. Roasting on an open fire is far from the only option, though. Fresh or reconstituted nuts combine beautifully in risottos, stews, soups, and purées. Chestnuts are challenging to grow—being fussy about soil, shade, and temperature. We tried them in Sumas, where walnuts, hazelnuts and fruit trees thrived, and they died within a couple of years. I'm guessing our rich, heavy loam was too wet for them. They are also tricky to store, as they are much more perishable than other nuts. Their high water content makes them prone to mold, and their thin shells mean than that fresh ones will dry unevenly and unsatisfactorily if not stored properly. I've had bad experiences getting them at the grocery store, and I recommend ordering straight from the farm if possible. The Chestnut Growers of America have a directory for commercial growers in the US and Canada, and many do mail order. For example, Chestnutsonline.com sells fresh and dried nuts, flour, and gluten-free baking mixes from their farm in Ridgefield, WA, on the Oregon border north of Portland. They hold farm tours during National Chestnut Week (who knew?) in October. If you have a windfall supply of fresh nuts, they can be refrigerated in a plastic bag for a couple of weeks or peeled and frozen. Dried chestnuts do keep well.

Foragers take note: the lovely Northwest native horse chestnut tree is a different family and produces nuts that look similar but are only marginally edible and are toxic when eaten raw. They are not a useful substitute. If you have the space for at least two large trees (chestnuts need a pollinator), and the right conditions, you can buy stock and get detailed information from Washington Chestnut Company in Everson, WA: washingtonchestnut.com

chicory

C I C H O R I U M   E N D I V A   V A R .   C R I S P A

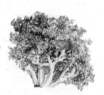

The nomenclature for chicory and its relatives is confusing, to say the least. Common names have undergone strange transmutations as they traveled from European kitchens, so that the Brussels (or Witloof) chicory they serve in Brussels is better known here as Belgian endive, and the French *chicorée frisée* is sold in the US as curly endive. The glamorous red radicchios are also chicories (or endives), as is escarole. Heirloom American recipes calling for "succory" also mean chicory. Check your recipe carefully for clues before you harvest or shop.

For purposes of this book, chicory is a curly- or toothy-leaved, loose-headed plant with a characteristic bitter tang. It is highly regarded as a salad green, and I think it's even better cooked. The garden plants are robust and hardier than lettuce, although constant rain discourages them. If you give them some shelter from the rain, they will thrive and sweeten through the first frosts of winter, resulting in better taste than you can buy. They keep well in a plastic bag in the refrigerator, with the added benefit that the bitterness moderates with time. The central leaves are paler and milder than the outer ones, allowing the cook to employ variations on the basic taste theme. (See also endive, escarole, and radicchio.)

collards

BRASSICA OLERACEA VAR. ACEPHALIA

Primitive members of the cabbage family, collards are among the most forgiving of vegetables. Cool-weather gardeners like them for their hardiness; they also hold up better in hot weather than their more refined cousins, which accounts for their starring role in Southern soul food. Even the most moribund-looking January collard may revive to produce sweet new greens in March, so don't be too quick to put them out of their misery. Here in Bellingham, the spring growth shows up at the farmers market as soon as it opens in April.

Since collards will live through most anything, you can hardly expect them to be delicate in flavor or texture. The leaves are thick and tough, and the flavor is assertive. Unlike a lot of greens, they respond well to long cooking and are excellent reheated. However, they are gaining fans in raw foods circles as a sturdy wrap covering, filling in for tortillas or rice noodles and holding up better than lettuce. I had one recently: early spring collard leaves wrapped around pumpkinseed pâté, avocado slices, salad greens and a whole lot of olive oil. It was delicious. They are an excellent vegetable source of calcium and are also high in vitamins A and C.

When shopping for collards, look for deep green—not yellowish—leaves and firm stems. Collards are never crisp, but they should not be limp and floppy.

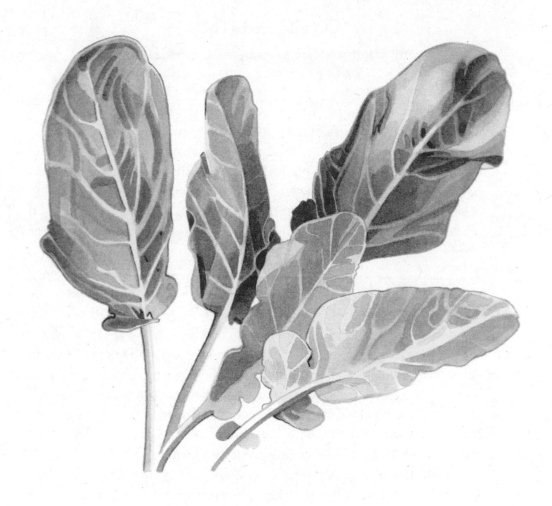

collards

· · · · · · · · · · · · · · · · · · · ·

corn salad

(field lettuce, lamb's tongue, mâche, feldsalat)

VALERIANELLA LOCUSTA

I used to find corn salad distressingly bland, but I've come around.
Its soft taste and texture make a good foil for more pungent winter
greens. This is a venerable and popular European market plant. It's
easy to grow—almost too easy at times, as its tiny seeds can spread
its range rapidly if you let it self-sow. I've used it as a winter ground
cover; it out-competes many of the weeds that gain footholds in
milder winters and is easy to dig under in the spring. Unbruised
plants will keep about a week under refrigeration.

dandelions

TARAXACUM OFFICINALE

In earliest spring, dandelion fanciers dot their yards with upended
flower pots to blanch the young growth of their favorite weed. Commercial seed, available from some catalogs, produces a slightly less
bitter green, but I doubt the difference is worth the expense. Seeds
marketed as Italian dandelion are actually a form of chicory, a different genus. Dandelion greens are used primarily in salads. They
are high in vitamin C among other nutrients, though not usually
eaten in such quantities as to make that a major consideration.
They don't keep well.

Although the roots have the stronger effect, the leaves are also
a diuretic (note the French common name, *pissenlit*), commonly
used in herbal tonics. Once the plant flowers, the leaves will be
too bitter to eat; however, the sunny flowers can be used to make
a traditional dessert wine.

endive

(Belgian endive, Witloof chicory)

CICHORIUM INTYBUS

. . . .

In this book, I use the name "endive" to mean the delicacy, resembling a pale, miniature head of romaine lettuce, that is served at outrageous prices in French restaurants. This chicon is produced by digging up the roots of the summer-sown plants in the fall, storing them in the dark, and harvesting the doomed, blanched shoots that result. A disciplined gardener can get an impressive supply for the cost of a packet of seed. That may be the only way you are likely to get enough endive to cook for company. Shoppers (unless cost is no object) are better off sticking to salads, where the leaves go further.

An endive chicon will keep for several days in the refrigerator. Don't wash it before storage, and keep it dark. The core is the most bitter. You can remove it with a paring knife if you want a milder flavor. (See also chicory.)

escarole

CICHORIUM ENDIVA

. . . .

A broad-leaved variety of chicory, escarole resembles a large, blowsy romaine. The flavor is similar to chicory, but the leaves are fleshier. Full-heart Batavian is the most common variety. The heart referred to is the blanched, delicious center, which is sweet with just enough bitter edge to be interesting. Escarole and chicory can be used interchangeably in most recipes. Like chicory, escarole tastes best after a frost, so Northwest-grown crops have a taste as well as environmental advantage over California and Florida imports. (See also chicory.)

florence fennel

(finocchio dolce)

FŒNICULUM VULGARE

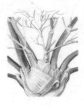

A lovely plant with feathery leaves and a fist-sized bulbous base, it resembles an elegant celery and is available in both green and bronze varieties. Both leaves and base are used, the former mostly in salads and as a garnish for fish and pork. The mild anise flavor adapts to a variety of treatments.

Shoppers should look for fresh-looking greens and firm, medium-sized bulbs. Try to buy whole plants rather than just the bulbs. You get more value, and you can judge the freshness by the leaves. Large, stringy bulbs can be deveined like celery. The bulbs keep fairly well refrigerated in a plastic bag; the greens should be used within a few days.

If you are growing fennel for the first time, locate it carefully, as it is very persistent and it gets big.

gobo

(burdock)

ARCTIUM SPP.

This is the same genus as cocklebur, the noxious weed whose prickly, tenacious seeds were the inspiration for Velcro. It is large, deep-rooted, and nearly indestructible once established, so I hesitate to recommend it as a garden plant unless you are far more organized and disciplined than I am. On the other hand, the taste is among the best of all winter roots: full and rich, with a bittersweet edge. Besides its culinary value, Japanese gobo (*Arctium lappa*) is widely taken in Japan to improve strength and virility, and the naturalized American varieties are used in a number of herbal remedies. You often can find gobo in Asian markets and specialty groceries.

The dark brown root is the most important culinary part. It is long—up to 18 inches—and slender; you will need to dig it, not pull it. Although the young leaves are sometimes used as a green, I find them unpleasantly hairy and bitter.

good king henry
(Mercury, Lincolnshire spinach, poor man's asparagus)
CHONOPODIUM BONUS HENRICUS

Like sorrel and mint, this heirloom potherb is welcomed as one of the first herbs of spring. A member of the goosefoot family, as is its tasty wild relative, lambsquarters, it has thickish arrow-shaped leaves that can be steamed or mixed with milder flavors in salads. The "poor man's asparagus" name comes from the early spring shoots, which can be picked and steamed.

hamburg parsley
(turnip-rooted parsley)
PETROSELENIUM CRISPUM VAR. TUBEROSUM

A variety of parsley grown for its root, which looks like a small skinny parsnip and has a nice mild parsley taste, it deserves more notice than it gets, being unfussy in the garden and very hardy. It is easier to harvest than the deep-rooted parsnip (though less productive) and much easier to clean than celeriac, and can be substituted for both in many recipes. It's very good in stews and hearty soups and has many uses in folk medicine. The strong-flavored leaves can be substituted, sparingly, for regular parsley.

Gardeners can leave the plants in the ground through the winter and harvest as needed. Shoppers should look for crisp, solid roots and store them like carrots. They will keep for a week or two.

jerusalem artichokes

(sunchoke, topinambour, earth apple)

H E L I A N T H U S   T U B E R O S E M

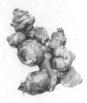

If you grow Jerusalem artichokes, you probably have more than you can eat. These prolific members of the sunflower family (the name "Jerusalem" is probably a corruption of the Italian *girasole*, "sun-turning") are among the hardiest of vegetables, surviving and multiplying through summer droughts and winter blizzards. John Goodyer, a young English botanist who received two tubers of the New World curiosity in 1617, reported that they increased a hundredfold in his garden. "I stocked Hampshire," he noted in his journal. Lately they are experiencing a modest renaissance, and varieties developed during their European diaspora are making their way back to North America.

This is good because Stampede, the only type I had seen until recently, is pale, knobby, and just plain funny looking. (Just recently I saw a fellow shopper recoil dramatically at the sight of them in the produce section. I gave my best jchoke pep talk, but she wouldn't even touch one, let alone buy it.) More to the point in the kitchen, the bumps make them hard to clean and next to impossible to peel. Fuseau varieties, which come in red and white skinned versions, are much smoother. They are also somewhat less productive, but that's not a problem with such a prolific plant. The Red Fuseau is the closest I have seen to the type much appreciated in Turkey as the Earth Apple (Yerelmasi). I thought the Fuseau flavor was a bit richer as well.

Jerusalem artichokes are a boon to dieters and diabetics because they are low in calories and they store their carbohydrates in the form of inulin. (For some people, however, they also have a beanlike tendency to produce impressive intestinal sound effects.) They have a sweet, clean taste, somewhat reminiscent of a water chestnut.

They do not keep as well as potatoes, and they need to be refrigerated, so gardeners shouldn't harvest more than a week's worth at a time.

oikostreecrops.com is a good source of information.

kale

(chou frisé)

BRASSICA OLERACEA VAR. CAMPESTRIS;
BRASSICA NAPUS

. . . .

Kale is the reason I originally wrote *Winter Harvest*. Under Binda Colebrook's tutelage, I grew some handsome plants and marveled as they survived everything a Sumas winter could dish out. The only trouble was I didn't know what to do with them. In researching recipes, I learned that kale was once so ubiquitous that in Scotland "kailyard" was synonymous with garden. One of the most popular garden varieties, Siberian, gives another clue as to its winter hardiness. Kale can handle heat as well as cold, and it shows up in Southern European, Middle Eastern, and North African dishes as well.

In the 20 years since the first edition, kale has moved much closer to the vegetable mainstream, and more varieties are commonly available. Basically there are two species of kale, and three main visual types.

Siberian kale, *Brassica napus,* is most common garden variety and, in my experience, the easiest to grow in winter. It gets big. The one in my alley planter was pushing four feet this spring and took a hatchet to cut down when it finally went to seed in early June. The leaves are frilly and bluish green, and it is the type most often used for salads as well as cooking. Russian kale, red Russian kale, and similar *napus* varieties are also notably cold hardy. Their leaves are more open and less frilly though still irregular.

Siberian and Russian kales will reliably overwinter down to at least 20°F as long as they get a good start before the heavy frosts hit in your area. I have dug down through snow to get at them and had them for dinner that same night. They are sweeter after a light frost; if you want them for salad, that's the best time. After a really hard freeze, the leaves get a bit tattered and not so attractive for eating raw.

Brassica oleraceae includes the multinamed Tuscan Black Palm Kale, Lacinato, Dinosaur Kale, or simply Toscana, as well as collard greens. They have savoyed (a lot of catalogs call them dimpled) leaves, and in my experience a stronger flavor. They are also the most heat tolerant and bolt resistant of kales. Kale soup recipes from Portugal and Italy have these varieties in mind.

Versatile in the kitchen, kale can be used sparingly as a raw salad green, more abundantly as a cooked green, lasagna ingredient, pizza topping, soup green, in pasta, or quickly broiled.

Kale is famously high in phytonutrients, leading many people to feel as though they *should* be eating it regularly, even when they don't know how to prepare it. It is also an excellent source of vitamins K, A, and C. Another nutritional plus is that it lends itself to low-fat cooking treatments. Although it's great in soup with bacon or sausage, it's also just fine steamed with no fat at all.

kiwi

ACTINIDIA DELICIOSA

hardy kiwi

ACTINIDIA ARGUTA

. . . .

I didn't consider kiwi for the first edition because I just assumed they were tropical fruit in the manner of guavas. But then my friends Carolyn Dale and Tim Pilgrim, whose trellised kiwis provide summer shade in their beautiful Bellingham backyard, gave me a boxful in November. I learned they are picked green in early fall and need at least a month to fully ripen. Those kiwis were so much tastier than any I have had on a caterer's tray that I realized I've been missing out.

My other revelation a few years back was a taste test of hardy kiwi at Cloud Mountain Farm. These are not the familiar fuzzy kind but grape-sized, smooth-skinned fruit that concentrates all of a large kiwi's flavor into a much smaller space. As the name implies, the hardy vines are cold tolerant and also as exuberant as wisteria once they get going. However, they are a long-term project for gardeners, as they commonly take at least four years to begin bearing in quantity. Harvests are also vulnerable to blossom-killing early frosts in colder regions; the vines will endure, but you may not get fruit. Like raspberries, they bear on second-year wood, so pruners need to watch what they're doing.

kohlrabi

(Hungarian turnip)

BRASSICA OLERACEA CAULORAPA

This is more a cool-weather crop than a real winter stalwart, at least where I live. It keeps and travels well, however, and its flying saucer appearance is good for a smile. Despite the Hungarian turnip name, it's not a turnip, but a closer cousin to broccoli and cauliflower. The edible portion is not a root but an above-ground swollen stem. It can be eaten raw or cooked (but not overcooked) in most recipes calling for broccoli or turnips. I also read a blog post from a cook who uses it as a more digestible substitute for green peppers. The purple and green varieties taste the same to me.

Look for firm, medium-sized globes with a healthy sheen. If they are pitted or spotty, they've been around too long, and the really large ones may have a tough core, although Territorial Seeds says its big Superschmeltz variety stays crisp all the way through. You have to peel them; a paring knife works better than a potato peeler.

leeks

ALLIUM AMPELOPRASUM VAR. PORRUM

Leeks are among the oldest cultivated vegetables, taking their name from the Old English word *leac*, or "plant." English kitchen gardens were once called leek gardens, just as their Scotch counterparts were called kailyards. In folklore, leeks are most associated with the Welsh, who wear them in their hats on St. David's Day, and consume them in cock-a-leekie soup, among other dishes.

Although market gardeners find that giant leeks sell the best, the smaller ones taste better. Pencil-sized leeks are sweeter and milder than green onions and make a fine addition to an antipasto plate. I keep a batch of small ones, stunted by the calculated neglect of not thinning them, for mid-winter green-onion substitutes. Medium-sized ones are best for side dishes and cooked salads. I use the monsters in vichyssoise or purées.

The white shaft of a leek is produced by hilling soil up around the growing plant to blanch it. It has a milder flavor than the green part, so the more subtle the dish, the less green you should use. The outer leaves are too stringy for good eating but can be added to stocks. A mid-winter leek can look weather-beaten and still taste fine, but you should discard any with a yellow or brown tinge to the stalk.

If you move a few overwintered leeks to the flower border in spring, they will shoot up 4 or 5 feet and reward you with dramatic balls of white or lavender flowers in July, and you can save your own seed for the following year.

lettuce

LATUCA SATIVA

With a bit of planning and perhaps a cold frame, most Pacific Northwesterners can have garden lettuce from April into December. I've been amazed how hardy these tender-looking plants can be. It must be fun to breed lettuce as well, judging by the ever-proliferating varieties available from seed catalogs. I've also eaten some fine salads from the progeny of overwintered lettuces that went to seed in my summer garden and propagated themselves. Still, winter lettuces endure the cold months but can't be expected to grow much, so this is not the time to plan a big home-grown Caesar salad. A mixture of lettuce, spinach and corn salad is a more realistic expectation for mid-winter.

If your problem is oversupply—a lot of sad looking lettuce that is about to bolt in early spring—you can substitute lettuce for Chinese cabbage and other mild greens in stir-fries and soups. These uses have ample precedent. Julia Child discusses lettuce cookery in *Mastering the Art of French Cooking*, and grilled romaine recipes are showing up on a number of foodie websites.

mushrooms

. . . .

I grew up foraging for mushrooms and still take extra pleasure in finding urban patches. (A local car wash used to have crops of spring morels in its planting strip, though I haven't seen them lately.) I love the thrill of the hunt, the chance to be in the woods, the euphonious names—Questionable Stropharia, *Lactaria deliciosa*—and the subtle fragrances and astounding variety of shapes and sizes. After all that, actually eating them could seem anticlimactic, but I love the tastes too—raw, sautéed, baked and pickled. For the less straightforward identifications, I like the process of making spore prints and checking the results with my trusty copy of *The Savory Wild Mushroom*.

A couple of years ago in Whatcom County, we had one of those Western Washington non-summers, where it rained pretty much straight through from May to September. The silver lining was that it was an epic year for chanterelles. My friend and neighbor Bob Holmgren dried so many that he made batches of chanterelle flour as Christmas presents. What a treat. Should you have a similar bounty, he says it's easy. Dry the mushrooms thoroughly and use a coffee grinder to reduce them to a powder. That's it. I used some of my portion to make the most seductive béchamel I have ever added to a lasagna.

I do buy criminis and portabellas. Other than that, I just can't get myself to pony up the prices charged for wild-harvested chanterelles, morels, and boletes. If I don't forage my own, I do without. Another option is to buy one of the many home mushroom kits sold by Fungi Perfecti, among others. My experience with these has been mixed, but it's fun and worth a try.

Novice mushroom gatherers should get a good guidebook, and go out with an expert before venturing on their own. Even the best photos and drawings are not a substitute for being with someone who can show you the difference between, say, a fried chicken mushroom (delicious and safe) and a livid entoloma (also tasty, I've been told, but poisonous). Several species will ruin your day, and a few, notably the Amanita verna (common name: Destroying Angel) can kill you.

mustards
BRASSICA SPP.

There is a bewildering assortment of garden mustards, not to mention the wild types found in nearly every vacant lot and alley. Since these brassicas crossbreed with enthusiasm and self-sow with abandon, there is no telling what hybrids will crop up in your garden next spring. Students of particular cuisines will want to track down specific types. Garden stores and catalogs are getting more and more sophisticated in their offerings, but the overlap of common names makes it hard to be positive what you are planting. Territorial Seed Company has a good selection, and I recommend their catalog as a place to begin your researches.

My personal culinary taxonomy divides mustards into Southern and Asian, and I usually grow some of each. "Southern mustards" are the large, strong-flavored types generally found in the supermarket next to the collards. They need longer cooking, preferably in the company of a ham hock or a bit of bacon. In my garden, tyfon, which is also grown as a forage crop for livestock, fills the bill. I harvest some in midsummer for big cooking greens and some in fall for winter salads.

Asian mustards (and cabbages—the distinction is often academic in the kitchen) come in amazing variety—*mizuna, santoh,* bok choy, *tat soi,* green-in-snow, golden streaks, and ruby streaks and on and on. These vary a lot. Some are grown as much for the stem as for the leaves and are very mild in flavor. Others are nearly all leaf and intensely "green" in taste. Some are very peppery, some hardly at all. Most of them are easy to grow, and many are beautiful enough for a place in the ornamental garden. They make an excellent introduction to winter gardening, since they are easy and versatile.

Freshness is the key when buying mustard greens. The small frilly types spoil quickly; the big tough ones will keep quite a while, but they quickly lose their sweetness and become merely hot and harsh.

nettle

URTICA SPP.

. . . .

Most Northwesterners were nonplussed when nettle soups first appeared at fancy prices in some Seattle restaurants. The ubiquitous stinging nettle is probably second only to the equally ubiquitous slug on the local hate list. However, cooking eliminates the sting, and nettles have a long and honorable history as a potherb. In his 18th-century tour of the Hebrides, Samuel Johnson reports sitting down to a bowl of nettle soup served on a cloth made of nettle fiber. And on my 2010 trip to Romania, I received an enthusiastic description of a favorite local nettle soup recipe.

Northwest Native people made fishing nets and blanket warps out of nettle fiber—which should be a clue to one culinary drawback. Because the stalks become very fibrous indeed, nettles should be picked young, and only the leaves should be used in cooking. I use plants no more than six inches high for omelets and other greens. You have a little more leeway if you are making a purée.

Nettles are an early spring rather than a real winter plant. The late fall growth is too coarse to eat, and the first frost mows it down. But by late February in a mild year, the first new shoots can be found in city lots as well as rural woods. Keeping a patch trimmed will encourage tender new growth throughout the year, but I think they taste best in springtime. Wear rubber gloves for picking and cleaning.

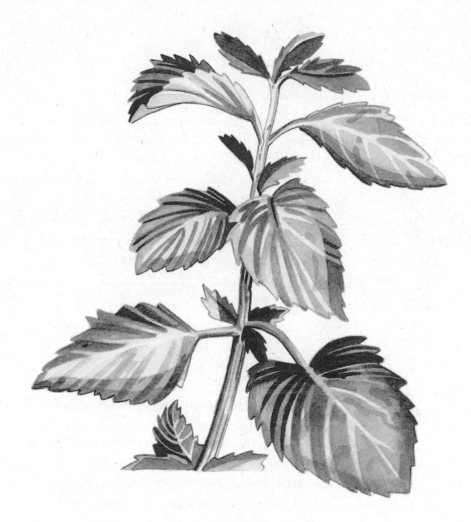

nettle

. . . .

orach

(mountain spinach)

A T R I P L E X   H O R T E N S I S

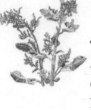

A member of the goosefoot family, orach is an annual relative of another heirloom vegetable, Good King Henry. It has big, thin savoyed leaves that resemble spinach in looks and flavor. Red, yellow, and screaming neon magenta-leaved forms are grown as ornamentals. They can reach five feet in height and reseed with ease, making them popular with edible landscapers. The seeds are also favored by the western goldfinch, Washington's beautiful state bird. It is not fully hardy but will take light frosts, and self-seeded plants get going by April where I live.

parsnips

P A S T I N A C A   S A T I V A

The introduction of the potato to Europe in the 18th century ended the parsnip's reign as the premier winter root. Until then, they were a northern staple, especially during Lent in Catholic countries, where they provided the bulk if not all the savor of the missing meat. Parsnips are not as versatile in the kitchen as the blander spud, and their long roots and even longer growing season make them more trouble in the garden. Another strike against them in the commercial world is that they don't taste their best until they have been through a freeze. The ones in the grocery store may therefore be pasty-tasting imitations of the real thing.

Nevertheless, I have come to appreciate them more in recent years, even though I no longer have the garden room to grow them. (That space is reserved for scorzonera, which is harder to find in the store.) I get them at the farmers market, where I appreciate the

choice between small parsnips the size of their carrot cousins—
great for slicing thin and roasting with some seasoned salt—and the
monsters destined for purées and stews. The big ones keep fairly
well; small ones should be used right away or they will go limp.

pears

(European: comice, bosc, highland, seckel
Pyrus communis
(Asian: chojuro, atago, Korean giant)
Pyrus serotina

The classic Bartlett pear has ripened and gone by the time cool
weather comes. In good years, Bartletts rival zucchini in their
abundance, and the slightest expression of interest will get you
bags of fruit from overwhelmed backyard growers. I like to dry
slices and add them to apple crisps and pies. But winter shoppers
will find fresh Comices, Boscs, Seckels and other varieties that keep
clear into spring. These are also, for my money, the most flavorful and succulent of all pear types. The proliferation of Asian pear
varieties in the last decade has added new names to the cool season
list. With all these choices, you can pick textures from crunchy
Atagos to buttery Comice, and flavors ranging from an almost
apple tartness to an ultrasweet Seckel (aka sugar pear).

If I had room, I would grow Comice for its beauty, taste, keeping qualities, and its magical affinity for a sliver of Roquefort
cheese. If you grow your own—and many old-country places come
equipped with a few old pear trees—pay careful attention to the
harvesting instructions for your variety. Some ripen on the tree;
others must be picked green and ripened in storage.

potatoes

SOLANUM TUBEROSUM

· ·

Potatoes wax and wane in trendiness, depending on whether complex carbs or low carb are the buzzwords of the moment. But they are just too good and too versatile to go away. Since the first edition of *Winter Harvest*, varieties that were little-known outside of specialty catalogs have gone mainstream. Yukon Golds and French fingerlings are in the bins at my local supermarket. Still, home gardeners have an immense advantage in tailoring their crops to their favorite uses and growing lower-yielding varieties that have superior taste. Yukon Golds are a case in point. They are good, and their yellow flesh makes an especially attractive mashed potato, but Yellow Finns, which are less uniform in shape and are rarely seen in stores, taste even better.

A trip through a potato specialist's catalog—I favor Ronniger's— is also a chance to absorb some food history. Like the tomato, this New World crop has undergone amazing permutations in its global travels, and now comes back to us with varieties such as Valisa and Sieglinde from Germany, and Rote Erstling from Sweden, and La Ratte from Switzerland. Potatoes brought to the Northwest Coast by Spanish ships and by the traders of the Hudson's Bay Company were also taken up by Native American growers. The Makah Nation of the Olympic Peninsula has kept the Ozette fingerling variety going in backyard gardens since the 17th century, and it has recently been taken up by the Slow Food movement in an effort to expand its availability. Of course these don't even scratch the surface of potato diversity in its true home ground in the altiplano of Bolivia and Peru, where the International Potato Center maintains thousands of varieties, most of them grown only in South America.

quince

(ate)

CYDONIA OBLONGA

. . . .

The ornamental quince bushes common to Northwest yards and gardens sometimes set fruit that can be used in any quince recipe. One of my students brought me a delicious slice of quince pie, which her enterprising mom made from their backyard bush. (Thanks, Emily!) A culinary quince is taller—up to 20 feet—and bears a larger hard fruit, about the size and shape of an Asian pear. Quinces may be yellow, orange, or green on the outside, with hard grainy flesh ranging from white to orange. They ripen from late summer to fall and keep well.

Quinces must be cooked. They are high in pectin, and in North America they are generally relegated to jellies and preserves, but they have many other uses. In Iran and Turkey, where the species originated, they are added to slow-cooked lamb dishes and also used in Turkish delight. Quince paste, *ate de membrillo*, is a Mexican delicacy that comes in blocks in my local supermarket, often sold next to the panela cheese that is its excellent taste pairing. The slight astringency of cooked quince also will enliven a prosaic apple crisp or poached pear dessert.

Quinces have a pronounced and pleasant fragrance when ripe. Sniff before you buy or pick, handle gently, and refrigerate. Well-treated fruit will keep for several weeks.

raab

(brassica rapa ruvo)

RAPA, BROCCOLI RAAB

. . . .

This small brassica resembles a slender broccoli. It's easy to grow and less prone to rot during rainy autumns than broccoli itself. It may be the answer for gardeners with limited space and a passion for broccoli flavor. Common in Italian, especially Tuscan, recipes, it can be replaced by small broccoli or a mixture of broccoli and mustard greens. Stalks require peeling.

radicchio
(red chicory, treviso)
CICHORIUM INTYBUS

A truly beautiful plant, radicchio is a variety of the same species that is forced for Belgian endive chicon. The spectacular red-and-white-striped leaves look like small, festive lettuces. The Verona type is round; treviso is elongated, like a miniature romaine. It's popular in salads, either alone or mixed with milder greens for contrast in flavor and color, but I prefer it lightly cooked.

Radicchio is expensive, so choose each head carefully. It is not difficult to grow, although it's rather slow. Your garden heads may be looser and more strongly flavored than store-bought ones.

radishes
RAPHINUS SATIVUS

The small red salad radishes are not particularly hardy, but they are among the first crops to mature in spring. Some of the French icicle varieties are grown for their greens, but I haven't tried them.

Winter radishes, more common in Japanese and Chinese cooking, are usually represented in this country by daikon. They are used in a variety of ways, both pickled and fresh, and their thick white roots provide the image behind the Hawaiian insult "daikon leg." Black Spanish radishes, like daikon, grow large and keep well, their initially harsh flavor moderating in weeks or months of storage. I don't crave radishes enough to grow them, as they require vigilant protection against root-fly maggots, but I like pickled daikon and I intend to try black radish soon.

rampion
(Rapunzel, raperonzolo)
CAMPANULA RANUNCULUS

A venerable German salad green and root, which was the green craved by Rapunzel's mother in the eponymous fairy tale. Paul Zelinsky, the renowned children's book illustrator, grew his own as part the research for his retelling of the story, and documented the process on his website: paulozelinsky.com/rapunzel.html.

I haven't grown or eaten this, but it is a cool-weather crop with a long history, and tiny little seeds are available from specialty growers. The roots look a bit like small daikon and are commonly boiled and served with a béchamel. The greens, which look a lot like arugula and evidently share their tendency toward a nutlike flavor and variable hotness, are used in salads and in a traditional Italian dish of early spring, pansotti al preboggion, which is ravioli filled with wild greens and sheep's milk ricotta cheese.

rose hips
ROSA SPP.

Old-fashioned rugosa rose varieties have the largest, best-tasting hips. As an added benefit, the plants are immune to practically all the ills that more refined roses are heir to. The individual flowers are not as impressive as those of a tea rose, but the mass effect is pleasant. Rose hips have a nice tart taste and lots of vitamin C, but the fruit is small and seedy. They are most commonly used in teas and jellies, where the seeds can be strained out. Rose hips should be harvested before a heavy freeze. Be sure that the plants have not been sprayed with insecticides or fungicides. If the bugs can't eat it, you shouldn't.

rutabaga

(swedes, yellow turnips, neeps)

BRASSICA NAPUS VAR. NAPOBRASSICA

Rutabagas look similar to turnips and are treated interchangeably in many recipes, but to me, the rutabaga is closer in flavor to broccoli stems, Like broccoli, they are especially averse to overcooking and should not be boiled. If you are adding cubes to a soup or stew, save them for the last 10 minutes or so and keep the liquid to a simmer. Otherwise, steaming, roasting and baking work best.

Rutabagas range from the size of boiling potatoes clear up to grapefruit dimensions. I used to assume that the small ones would be sweeter and less fibrous, but after sampling some giants, harvested that day from my neighbors' garden, I've concluded that freshness, consistent water, and soil quality are the real determinants of taste. Also, the flavor improves after a light freeze, which may argue toward the bigger specimens that have been in the ground longer. They are easier than turnips to grow in size and quantity, being less vulnerable to the voracious root-fly maggot. Large or small, they should be sampled first to check texture and flavor, because a fibrous, overstrong morsel of rutabaga is nobody's treat. (A website footnote to a traditional Scotch recipe for Bashed Neeps, often served with haggis, claims you can use the leftovers as mortar for household repairs.)

salsify

(oyster plant, barba di becco)

TRAGOPOGON PORRIFOLIUS

. . . .

A popular 19th-century root, salsify is benefiting from the vogue for specialty vegetables. All simple treatments—steamed, sautéed, puréed, creamed, or glazed—are good and easy, once you get past the chore of peeling the hairy, wiggly roots. (The Italian name *barba di becco* means "billy goat beard.") Escoffier favored a marinade of olive oil and lemon juice, before deep-frying them. Don't expect a true oyster taste, but the flavor is pleasantly different from that of parsnips and carrots: fuller, I guess you could say, and not so sweet. Salsify and scorzonera (below) are similar enough in taste and texture to be interchangeable in recipes.

Salsify is easy to grow, although very slow, and it is extremely hardy. You do need loose soil (see growing tip for scorzonera, below), since the roots are long and slender. They can be left in the ground through the winter, but if you want to harvest before the soil freezes hard, the roots will keep for weeks in a plastic bag in the refrigerator.

scorzonera

(picridie, viper's grass, winter asparagus)

SCORZONERA HISPANICA

. . . .

I just love scorzonera, and now that I've relocated a source for seeds (Stellar Seeds; see Resources) I intend to have lots of it. I also have a deep planter bed with sandy soil, another requisite for a manageable crop of this unusual-looking, rich-tasting root. Scorzonera is a long, thin, black-skinned root, often called the black oyster plant for its resemblance to salsify, though it is a different genus. It can be tricky to harvest without breaking. (One suggestion is to grow it in deep tubs of sandy soil. Then you can just upend the tub at harvest time and fish out the roots.) Like Jerusalem artichokes, scorzonera is a member of the sunflower family and is rich in inulin, which is good news nutritionally, but which spells intestinal gas for some people who have trouble digesting it. It's probably best not to combine your first experience with a first romantic dinner. Also like jchokes, scorzonera can go quickly from just right to overcooked, especially when boiled. Roasting and sautéing are safer bets as you get to know their quirks. Roasted scorzonera with a bit of olive oil or butter and a squeeze of lemon will demonstrate why many people compare the flavor to artichokes.

Don't be put off if the roots are a bit sticky; that's natural and will come off with washing, but they should not be limp.

sorrel

RUMEX SPP.

Members of the buckwheat family, wild sorrels are everywhere. Even the more refined French garden type is easy to grow—in fact, it's hard to get rid of once established.

Sorrel doesn't keep well. Use it the day it's bought or picked, and cook very lightly if at all; overcooked sorrel is mushy. (Don't use an aluminum or cast-iron pan, or the leaves will turn an unappetizing blackish brown.)

If you cut back rank summer growth in September, you will get a nice new crop of fall leaves that will keep producing until a heavy freeze. Then the spring crop will be up with the daffodils, providing wonderful, bright-tasting salads when you need them most. Another salad resource with similar flavor is oxalis, in either its green or reddish-leaved form.

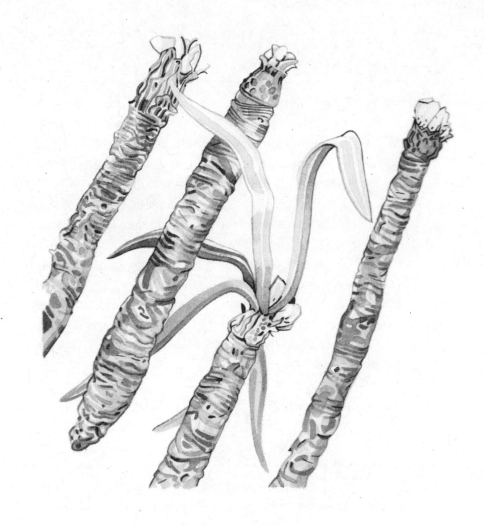

scorzonera

spinach

SPINACEA OLERACEA

Better to buy frozen spinach than some of the bedraggled muddy bunches that turn up in markets in winter. Better yet to grow your own. Winter-hardy spinaches usually have savoyed or semi-savoyed leaves—Bloomsdale Savoy is the old campaigner; Winter Giant, a newer variety. Unlike spring and summer crops, which are closely planted so the plants can provide each other a bit of shade and cooler air, winter spinach crops need wider spacing and as much light as you can find. They can withstand cold temperatures, bounding back in spring even after a hard freeze, but they don't like to be clammy and damp for weeks on end.

You would need a much bigger garden than mine to make spinach lasagna in February, but the individual leaves, carefully harvested for a winter salad, will be the sweetest, richest, best spinach you ever have tasted.

squash

CUCURBITA SPP.

In the first edition, I felt the need to make a real pitch for winter squash, because I was only a recent convert myself and I knew so many other squash haters. My recent informal survey—consisting mostly of talking to my fellow teachers at lunch—indicates that this has changed. More and more people seem to have experienced spicy squash soups, squash ravioli and gnocchi, or little Acorns or Delicatas stuffed with all manner of fillings from veal to vegan. Japanese, African, and Mediterranean cuisines all make inventive and flavorful use of these New World vegetables.

It's good for me that more squash varieties are available in stores and farmers markets, since I no longer have room to grow more than one hill. That has also forced me to choose my favorite: it's Kabocha.

Home gardeners should note that, unlike most storage crops, squashes like a bit of warmth as well as dryness. I cure mine on top of the kitchen cabinets. Also, despite the old line about the frost on the pumpkin, it's better to bring them in before a freeze. Most squashes store well, but some hold their flavor much better than others. Delicatas, pumpkins, acorn, and spaghetti squashes are all close relatives of summer squashes like zucchini and patty pans, and they are best eaten within a month or two at most. They get blander and more fibrous as winter wears on. Buttercups, Butternuts, Hubbards, and Japanese Kuris and Kabochas belong to a different species (moschata); they stay sweet and smooth much longer.

sweet potatoes and yams
(batata, camote)
IPOMOEA BATATAS

I always hated sweet potatoes until I learned that they go better with soy sauce than with melted marshmallows. Since then I've become a devotee, expanding my experiments into roasting, soups, pies, tempura, and even biscuits. Last time I included them despite their non-local provenance, because they are such wonderful keepers and a great foil to strong-flavored winter roots and greens. Now Maritime Northwest locavores can take a shot at growing their own. Territorial Seeds offers slips, and a number of local gardeners have had success. That being said, the consensus is that local crops aren't as sweet as the ones grown in Southern heat, and I don't expect to see them as a local market crop anytime soon. Grocery store sweet potatoes and yams are just different varieties of the same plant. I buy the orange, or garnet, "yams" because I like the color better, but I'd be hard pressed to distinguish the taste. A bright purple variety, called 'uala, is popular in Hawaii, where it is used to make a truly neon-colored cheesecake. The true yam (*Dioscorea* spp.) is a large starchy tropical root that tastes more like a potato.

swiss chard

(spinach beet, silver beet, perpetual spinach)

BETA VULGARIS VAR. CICLA

· ·

Chard is prolific and tough, probably the most reliable winter green in terms of cool-weather production, and overwintered plants will stage a welcome comeback in early spring. Provençal and Spanish cuisines make especially good use of chard, but it is valued from Mexico to Russia. (Oddly enough, I've yet to run across any specifically Swiss recipes for chard.) French cooks in particular have created a number of recipes that focus on the stems rather than the leaves, and varieties such as Lucullus and Fordhook Giant have broader stems to accommodate those treatments. Breeders have also had fun with color, developing varieties from gold to red to magenta, which look beautiful in the garden before they head to the kitchen.

Give some thought to matching the chard to the recipe. New spring growth is fine with brief cooking and light seasoning, and very young leaves are good in salads. Big tattered December leaves had better go into soup or lasagna. Chard leaves can be stuffed like cabbage, with the same fillings.

Chard keeps a few days in the refrigerator, and stalks can be saved for a week or so, until you have accumulated enough for a separate recipe.

turnips

(navet)

BRASSICA RAPA

. . . .

Turnips have been cultivated since prehistoric times, and their sturdiness has made them a vegetable of last resort, to be fed to the stock when times are good and brought to the table when times are bad. Carved and lighted, they were also the precursor of the jack-o'-lantern pumpkin. Turnips are particularly esteemed in Japan, where they are commonly pickled or added to soups, and France, where they accompany meats. Julia Child praised the "wonderful vegetable" that "wants and needs to absorb butter or meat fats." Small, quick-growing types are steamed, sautéed, or pickled. Big, winter keepers are best for stews and purées.

Root-fly maggots just love turnips, and it takes some work to outwit them. I don't often go to the trouble. If I did, I would seek out the Japanese varieties such as hakurei or the bright red hidabeni.

citrus fruits

· ·

Oranges, lemons, and limes are never really in season in the Pacific Northwest, but they are at their best during our winter. Actually, thanks to my potted Meyer lemon tree, I do have homegrown citrus a good portion of the year, plus heaven-scented blossoms every Thanksgiving. When I need more than I can grow, I buy organically grown citrus, especially when recipes call for grated peel. Government-authorized safe consumption levels for the many chemicals used on citrus crops, which are already more tolerant of toxics than they should be, are based on the fruit inside, not the peel that actually receives the spray. If a recipe calls for the juice and not the rind, I freeze the squeezed out remains and save them for a time when I need peels. Besides saving money and making the most out of an item that was likely shipped from far away, another benefit of this technique is that frozen peels are much easier to grate.

tomatoes

· ·

Canned tomatoes usually are the best choice for winter cooking. Fresh ones, even when they aren't pale orange and hard as baseballs, are nearly always a disappointment. Plum tomatoes are relatively low in moisture and hold their texture better canned than do beefsteak types. I don't like to can, so I freeze and dry any surplus tomato harvest.

Freezing tomatoes is ridiculously easy and preserves true fresh tomato taste, though at the expense of texture. Just wash some perfect ripe tomatoes, dry thoroughly, and pop into the freezer in a plastic bag—no blanching or peeling necessary. Remove from the freezer half an hour before you need them. They will look just like fresh tomatoes and feel like icy little bowling balls. Remove skin by placing them in a bowl of warm water for about 30 seconds. The skin, which toughens when frozen and is best kept out of recipes, will crack and then slip smoothly off.

The thawed tomatoes will be watery and mushy. You can't slice them for a salad, but they are just fine—better than anything you can buy in a Pacific Northwest winter—in a blender salsa or a lightly cooked soup.

Dried tomatoes are easy to make at home if you have a food dryer or a gas oven. My climate seldom provides the sunshine needed to dry them outside in the classic fashion. Take firm, ripe tomatoes. Wash and dry them, then slice into rounds about a quarter-inch thick. Place on drying racks over a steady, gentle heat source. Dry until stiff and very chewy (about two days in my food dryer). Pry the translucent slices off the rack. They can be kept in a sealed plastic bag or, more glamorously, in a jar of olive oil with some sliced garlic and a few leaves of basil.

They are great in stews and soups, as a last-minute addition to sautéed leeks or broccoli, on pizzas, in steamed rice, and on sandwiches. They are hard to cut with a knife; use scissors instead. The flavored olive oil is perfect in salad dressings.

eggs

. . . .

Getting eggs used to be simple, in a way. After we raised the peeping little fluffballs under lights, protected them from their many predators, culled out the roosters that made it through the sexing process, grew greens for their enjoyment, hunted up healthy laying mash for them, and mucked out under their roosts, all we had to do was go out to the chicken house in the afternoon and gather the designer shades of green, blue, and brown eggs and decide what to do with them. These days I have way too many decisions to make at the store: white or brown? vegetarian diet or not? free-range but non-local or caged but local? organic feed? Much of this depends on budget and individual priorities, so I will stick with what I know, which is what makes a chicken happy and what kinds of eggs taste best.

Chickens are omnivores, and they want to be outside in the sunshine, taking dust baths and chasing bugs. The "vegetarian diet" promo on many cartons is to reassure us that they are not risking contamination by being fed ground-up remains of other chickens and even less-savory animal parts. But a free-range chicken will get about 30 percent of its diet from animal, meaning worm and insect, protein. That's one reason eggs from pasture-raised hens have thicker shells, brighter yolks, and denser whites than those from confined birds. They whip up faster for superior angel cakes and soufflés, they poach in compact little bundles, they make brilliant yellow scrambled eggs, and they taste just wonderful. It also turns out they are better for us, being lower than factory-farmed eggs in fat and cholesterol, higher in vitamins, and rich in those Omega 3 fatty acids that have us gulping down fish oil capsules. They are also inevitably more expensive, since agribusiness offloads the true costs of doing business onto future generations who have to live on the planet we are degrading.

meat

One thing that struck me when I looked back through the first edition with an eye to revising is how many recipes involved beef, chicken and pork, and how few used seafood. It's an indication of how closely the book represented my own situation. We raised our own livestock, and had more meat than we could use, so we seldom branched out. I couldn't make peace with the idea of killing young animals, so there are no lamb or veal recipes. Now that I'm off the farm, it's harder to find and afford meat that I feel good about, so the new recipes in this edition are mostly vegetarian.

None of our cows, chickens, turkeys, or hogs ever saw a feed lot or a slaughterhouse, and they got a minimum of commercial feed. Mostly they were part of the household economy. They ate the lush grass of the Sumas River bottom, table scraps, garden waste, windfall apples and pears. We collected the organic flour sweepings from Fairhaven Milling (thanks, Bill Distler!) and fed it to the pigs. The pigs also rooted their way through a patch of wild Sweet Cicely and picked up a faint fennel flavor. The Cornish cross chicks that swell to broiler size in eight weeks on a commercial farm took twice as long with us, and they were that much tougher and that much more flavorful as a result. I learned how to prepare and cook these leaner cuts of meat, experience that has come in handy now that marbling is suspect and grass-fed is in.

My homestead experience also influences my take on "food as politics." Though the environmental critiques of agribusiness in general and meat production in particular are devastating, I have a hard time imagining a sustainable farm economy that is entirely vegan. Our animals played so many roles on the homestead in addition to providing protein—eating scraps and prunings, fertilizing the garden and orchard, providing a bit of cash in the form of meat and milk sales, using the pasture that we lacked the time and equipment to convert to vegetable crops. And once we move our vision from vegan to vegetarian, we run into basic biology. If you want milk, you have to breed your cows and goats and produce babies. And eventually, dairy animals will get past their productive years. If you want eggs, you need chickens or ducks who will eventually be too old to lay. If we are serious about conserving resources, all those realities lead eventually to the kitchen. Hence the presence of meat recipes in a book that celebrates vegetables.

If we treated meat and dairy products as flavorful ingredients rather than the main course, and ate them occasionally rather than compulsively, we could move closer to an agriculture that is actually part of culture and that sustains us all.

sweeteners

. . . .

When it comes to thoughtful eating, there just isn't any free pass
on sweeteners. For example, recently trendy agave syrup has
its points, but it's refined, it's got about as much fructose as corn
syrup, and I just don't see any fields of Northwest agave to lower its
carbon footprint in my part of the world. Turbinado sugar or succanat, besides being expensive, is still sucrose, and it comes from far
away. Maple syrup is pricey and not produced anywhere near me,
though I've tasted some experiments with birch syrup from closer
to home. (I didn't like them much.) Honey can be locally produced,
but it doesn't work in all recipes. Individual dietary considerations
aside, it's more important to use sugar sparingly than to agonize
about its specific source. I'll admit to a major sweet tooth, and I'm
always looking for that "eat all you want for free" pass, but I know
I'm not going to find it.

For awhile I was thinking that the locavore choice might be
sugar beets. They were a big crop in Central Washington and Oregon when I was young, and I felt a chauvinistic pride in U&I beet
sugar instead of C&H, made from that foreign cane. Sugar beets are
making a modest Northwest comeback, and are being touted as a
biofuel, but they have major environmental issues. They are vulnerable to a number of pests and diseases, making them difficult to
grow organically on a large scale, and small-scale sugar production
is an unlikely concept. Furthermore, the favored commercial sugar
beet seed is a "Roundup Ready" GMO, which has sent neighboring
organic growers and environmentalists to court to stop its use.

In this book, I use a variety of sweeteners and look for ways to
limit the amount. Agave syrup is wonderful for tortes made with
puréed beets or carrots. It's thinner than honey and therefore easier to
work with, and unlike honey, it doesn't change its flavor when cooked
(presumably because it's already heated during processing). It's also

sweeter than white sugar, so you can use less. Succanat or date sugar both provide a warm, mild sweetness that doesn't overwhelm fruits and grains.

vegetable stock

. . . .

I've made some not-tasty vegetable stock in my time. I used to figure that pretty much any garden leftovers, plus some onion, would make a good broth. I was wrong. The wrong flavor balance can ruin the soup, especially soups designed to highlight mild vegetable flavors. Now that decent vegetable broth and vegetable bouillon mixtures are widely available, it's not necessary to make your own. However, every garden produces vegetables that are too grungy to serve up on their own but are ready to give their flavors to the pot. Here's a good basic combo. The lentils add a bit of depth that I like, especially in vegan dishes. Leave them out if you want a clearer, lighter stock. This freezes well, so make lots when the mood and the ingredients coincide.

an onion, roughly chopped
(I don't peel it. The skin adds color.)

2 medium leeks, white part only, chopped

2 carrots

2 cups of chopped garden greens. Chard and beet greens are good choices; lettuce is another possibility. Avoid the cabbage family except for maybe a bit of kale.

a handful of parsley

a bay leaf

2 celery sticks or 1/2 cup chopped celeriac (optional)

1/3 cup lentils

8 cups of water

Put all ingredients and the water in a large saucepan, bring to a boil. Reduce heat and simmer about 40 minutes. Strain, pushing the vegetables against the sides to collect those last bits of flavor. You can add salt to taste or wait and salt the soup when it's made.

a note on urban compost

I've lived most of my life in the country, with a compost pile close to hand. My parents grew up in town, but moved to a rural former dance hall before I was born. They brought the compost gospel back with them from a research sojourn in Switzerland in 1957. Every tidy kitchen garden in the tidy village of Coppet had a tidy and productive compost system. Ours at home was more laissez faire, a giant amorphous pile hidden in the woods behind a huge rhododendron, but it got the job done. The tight clay soil gradually loosened and transformed with its help. From childhood on, the only time I haven't made compost was in my Stanford dorm room.

On the farm, where we had the space and the materials to compost on a large scale, we really didn't need to (though we did anyway). The river bottom loam, augmented by the leavings of centuries of Native inhabitants who wintered there in pit houses, was six feet deep, black and rich. One of our thriftier neighbors used to come by every spring to collect our mole hills as potting soil.

Once I moved to town, I had much less space and much greater need. The soil is classic western Washington glacial clay in the back yard and, in the front, a barely cohesive powder that always reminds me of Hamlet's despairing description of the world as "this quintessence of dust." Water runs right off its sloping surface, worms find no sustenance, and the giant, glorious Norway maple next door forms dense root mats right up to the surface. The only place I have ever been unable to grow zucchini was in that insufficiently amended ground.

I didn't have the space, or the manure, for the farm system, nor the money for those spiffy circulating backyard drum models, but I needed to get going. The system I've evolved over the past few years is transforming the place, bucket by bucket. That front yard now produces blueberries, strawberries, peppers and squash in its few sunny patches, and I even have a small but productive peach tree.

I have three enclosed plastic bins. They sit side by side in a shady spot along the fence, and while not beautiful, they are unobtrusive. One is a pre-composter for the twiggier yard waste and for weeds that I want to make sure won't reseed or resprout in the garden. Materials go there to stay damp, begin to soften up, and for their seeds to sprout and die in the dark. Once or twice a year, I dump that container onto a tarp, put what's ready into the working compost and return the rest for another go. It takes about 20 minutes. The other two are the active composters. They are better ventilated and better tended. If I work it right, one is always nearing readiness, at least at the bottom layers, and the other is just getting going. So any time I want to transplant or fill a container, I have a shovelful or two of compost ready to go.

Lacking manure, my nitrogen source is coffee grounds, which the local stand bags up and leaves out by the dumpster for folks like me. Experiments by the Compost Specialists at Lane County Extension south of Portland, OR, have found that coffee grounds are more consistently effective than most manures in supplying and maintaining the heat it takes to make good compost quickly.

In the trials, when coffee grounds made up 25 percent of the volume of the compost pile, temperatures were sustained above 135°F for at least two weeks. Sustained heat makes faster, cleaner compost, as few pathogens and seeds can survive those temperatures for long. Compost Specialist Cindy Wise said that coffee grounds out-performed animal manures in raising and sustaining compost temperatures.

I used to worry that this influx of grounds would make the soil too acid for some of my plants, but it turns out the acid goes into the coffee we drink, and the grounds are more or less pH neutral.

You can also put grounds straight on the soil as mulch, but there are a couple of drawbacks. One is that your yard then tends to smell like stale coffee, especially after a rain, and another is that the nitrogen within is not directly available to the plants in that form. So it makes more sense to add them to the pile.

The rest of the piles comprise leaves, kitchen and garden scraps, and my shredded financial papers. It gives me great satisfaction to see old bills and bank statements turn into something unequivocally worthwhile.

gluten-free recipes

A note on **gluten-free** labeling. I want to err on the side of safety, so my aim in this book is to identify recipes that are gluten-free "by nature," meaning that one need not seek out gluten-free products to make them. That leaves out anything with canned soup stock, for example, since many brands contain gluten. I also eliminated dishes made with soy sauce, hot sauce, ketchup, and other prepared condiments, although gluten-free versions of all these are available. If you make your own stock, and know what to look for on the grocery shelves, the gluten-free options in this book expand considerably.

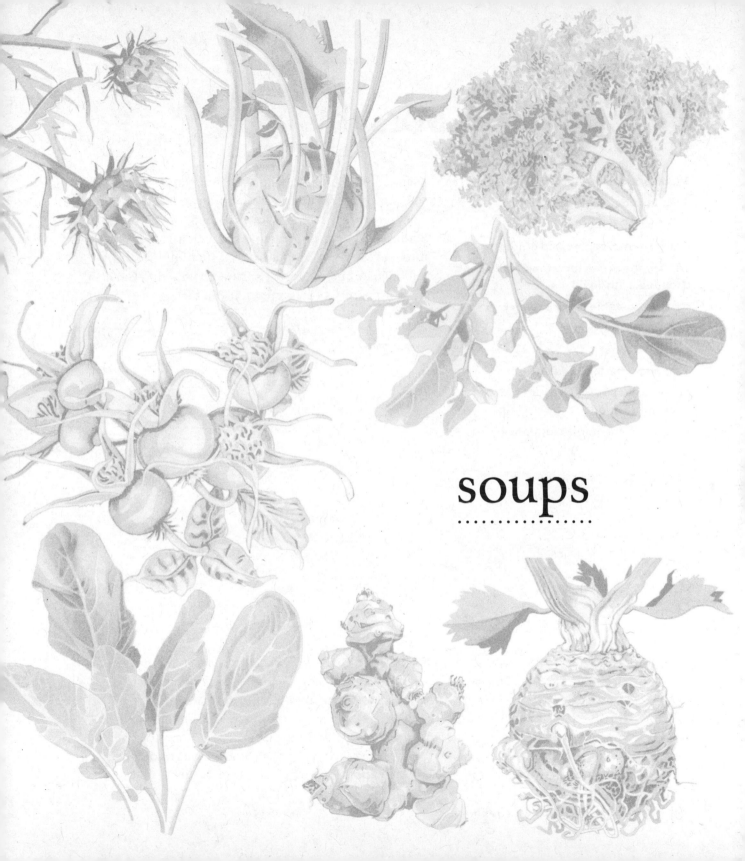

soups

borscht

3 tablespoons oil

1 medium onion, diced

3 or 4 carrots, grated

4 large beets, peeled and grated

one 15-ounce can tomatoes, roughly chopped, with liquid

4 cups vegetable stock or water

1/2 cup ketchup

salt and pepper

2 tablespoons lemon juice

1 tablespoon fresh dill or
1 teaspoon dried

sour cream for garnish (optional)

Heat oil in a big soup kettle. Add onion and sauté until soft. Add carrots and beets and sauté another 5 minutes. Add tomatoes, stock or water, ketchup, salt, and pepper. Bring to a boil, lower heat and simmer, and cook, covered, until vegetables are tender, about 40 minutes. Stir in lemon juice and serve hot, sprinkled with dill. Garnish with a spoonful of sour cream if you like.

Serves 6 as a first course or 4 as a main dish.

VEGAN

MY FRIEND KRISTIN BARBER FIRST SERVED ME THIS DELICIOUS VEGETARIAN BORSCHT MORE THAN 20 YEARS AGO. SHE WOULD MAKE IT BY THE GALLON FROM HER COUNTRY GARDEN AND THEN FREEZE IT. IT CONTAINS NO CABBAGE, AND THE TASTE IS FRESH AND BRIGHT. DON'T BE PUT OFF BY THE KETCHUP; MANY TRADITIONAL BORSCHT RECIPES CALL FOR TOMATO PURÉE, SUGAR, AND VINEGAR, WHICH ADD UP TO KETCHUP ANYWAY. YOU COULD SUBSTITUTE CHILI SAUCE FOR EXTRA ZIP. KRISTIN AND I ARE NOW NEIGHBORS IN OUR CURRENT STAGE OF LIFE AS TOWN DWELLERS, AND WE STILL TRADE RECIPES.

broccoli yogurt soup

1 **medium bunch broccoli**

3 **tablespoons butter**

1 **medium onion, coarsely chopped**

1/2 **cup chopped celeriac or Hamburg parsley**

4 **cups chicken broth**

2 **medium potatoes, peeled and cubed**

salt and pepper

3 **tablespoons chopped cilantro, divided**

1 **cup plain yogurt**

1 **cup milk or half-and-half**

Separate broccoli into florets. Peel stalks and cut into 1-inch lengths.

Melt butter in large saucepan. Add onion and celeriac or Hamburg parsley and toss to coat. Stir over medium heat until onion is tender. Pour in chicken broth. Add broccoli, potatoes, salt, pepper, and 2 tablespoons of the chopped cilantro. Simmer covered for 20 minutes or until broccoli is crisp/tender. Do not go all the way to soft; this dish is not a velvety bisque in texture.

Purée mixture and return to saucepan. In a separate bowl, mix together yogurt and milk or half-and-half, and add to soup. Warm gently, sprinkle with the remaining tablespoon of cilantro, and serve hot.

Serves 6.

VEGETARIAN

I LIKE THIS BETTER THAN STRAIGHT CREAM OF BROCCOLI SOUP. THE CILANTRO AND THE SLIGHT TANG OF YOGURT BRIGHTEN UP THE PROCEEDINGS. THE MOST IMPORTANT THING, AS WITH ANY BROCCOLI DISH, IS NOT TO OVERCOOK IT. HAMBURG PARSLEY, IF AVAILABLE, IS A MORE CONVENIENTLY SIZED ROOT THAN CELERIAC FOR A HALF-CUP QUANTITY. IF YOU USE REGULAR CELERY, GO FOR THE WHITE HEART MORE THAN THE GREEN STALK.

garbure

1/4 pound salt pork, chopped

1 medium onion, chopped

2 medium potatoes, peeled and chopped

2 leeks, chopped, with some green

1 rutabaga or turnip, peeled and chopped

1 large carrot, peeled and chopped

1 quart of water

half a green cabbage, sliced thin

3 cloves garlic, crushed

1 bay leaf

2 cups cooked white beans or favas, drained

salt and pepper

1/2 pound garlic sausage, sliced

1 sprig fresh thyme or 1/4 teaspoon dried

2 tablespoons chopped parsley

Render salt pork in large, heavy soup kettle. Add onion and sauté until soft. Add potatoes, leeks, rutabaga or turnip, and carrot and sauté another 2 or 3 minutes. Add water, cabbage, garlic, bay leaf, beans, salt, and pepper and bring to a boil. Lower heat and simmer about an hour or until vegetables are tender. Add sausage, thyme, and parsley and cook another 10 minutes.

Serves 6.

GARBURES ABOUND, AND A REALLY AUTHENTIC ONE, LIKE YOUR MOM'S FAVORITE SPAGHETTI SAUCE, IS UNLIKELY TO HAVE A WRITTEN RECIPE. ITS COMMON DENOMINATORS ARE BEANS, CABBAGE, CARROTS, AND LEEKS, AND SOME PORTION OF A PIG, WHETHER SAUSAGE OR BACON OR SALT PORK OR HAM HOCKS. THE DISH IS INDIGENOUS TO THE PYRENEES, CLAIMED BOTH BY THE BASQUES AND THE BÉARN REGION OF FRANCE. IT CAN BE MADE A DAY OR TWO AHEAD. I CANNOT VOUCH FOR THE AUTHENTICITY OF THIS VERSION, BUT IT IS EASY, ECONOMICAL, AND GOOD. I COOKED IT THE NIGHT BEFORE A SKI TRIP AND THEN REHEATED IT WHEN WE RETURNED HOME, COLD AND HUNGRY. ELIZABETH DAVID RECOMMENDS ADDING A FEW WHOLE ROASTED CHESTNUTS ALONG WITH THE CABBAGE.

basque soup

1/4 cup lard or olive oil

1 medium onion, chopped

1/2 pound pumpkin, peeled and cubed

1 medium cabbage, sliced

1/2 pound dried haricot beans or navy beans, soaked overnight and drained

2 cloves garlic, sliced

2 quarts stock or water

salt and pepper

Heat lard or olive oil in a large, heavy saucepan or soup pot. Add onion and brown. Add pumpkin, cabbage, beans, and garlic and cook briefly, stirring to coat the vegetables with oil.

Add stock or water, salt, and pepper, and bring to a boil. Lower heat to simmer and cook gently, covered, until beans are tender, about 2 hours. Adjust seasoning before serving.

Serves 6.

VEGETARIAN (IF NOT USING LARD), GLUTEN-FREE

THIS IS ADAPTED FROM ELIZABETH DAVID'S BOOK OF MEDITERRANEAN FOOD,
A GREAT SOURCEBOOK OF TRADITIONAL RECIPES (WITH TRADITIONALLY VAGUE
MEASUREMENTS). YOU MAY SUBSTITUTE OLIVE OIL FOR THE LARD; IT WON'T TASTE THE
SAME, BUT IT WILL BE GOOD. THIS SOUP HAS A ROBUST FLAVOR, AS YOU'D EXPECT,
AND WITH GOOD BREAD AND A SALAD, IT MAKES A COMPLETE MEAL.

caribbean cabbage soup

2 tablespoons light oil

1 teaspoon chopped fresh ginger

3 tablespoons minced onion

2 cups shredded green cabbage

6 cups water

1-1/2 cups diced unpeeled potatoes

1/2 pound raw shrimp, shelled and coarsely chopped (tiny shrimp can be used whole); if you have cooked shrimp instead, add them just before serving and heat through

salt and pepper

hot pepper sauce

1 tablespoon lemon juice

chives

Heat oil in a heavy saucepan or skillet. Add ginger and onion and sauté briefly. Add cabbage and sauté, stirring, until limp, about 3 minutes.

Bring water to a boil in a large kettle. Add potatoes and the cabbage mixture and simmer until potatoes are tender, about 15 minutes.

Add shrimp, salt, pepper, and a dash of hot pepper sauce and simmer another 5 minutes. Remove from heat and add lemon juice. Serve immediately, garnished with chopped chives.

Serves 4.

THIS SOUP MUST BE SERVED GOOD AND HOT. AND DON'T OVERCOOK THE CABBAGE. APART FROM THESE TWO POINTS, IT'S FOOLPROOF.

roasted cauliflower
hidden garlic soup

1 head garlic

4 tablespoons olive oil

4 cups cauliflower, in florets

1 cup chopped leeks, white part

1 medium potato, peeled and cubed

2 cups chopped celeriac

6 cups water or stock

bouquet garni of parsley, thyme, bay leaf and rosemary

1 teaspoon hot paprika

2 teaspoons lemon juice

2 tablespoons chopped Italian parsley

yogurt (optional)

Preheat oven to 400°F.

Slice off the top of the garlic head and pull and rub off as much of the skin as comes off easily. Put the head on a square of foil, big enough to cover, pour on about a tablespoon of olive oil and sprinkle with salt. Wrap the garlic up in the foil and bake until soft, at least 30 minutes.

Put the cauliflower on parchment paper or silicon sheet on a cookie tray. Pour a little olive oil on your hands and rub them onto the florets. Sprinkle with salt and spread onto one layer. Roast, checking often, until tender. It's OK if they color up.

Warm 2 tablespoons oil in a large pot. Sauté the chopped leeks over low heat until soft. Do not let them brown. Add potatoes, celeriac, stock or water, cauliflower, and bouquet garni. Squeeze the roasted garlic out of the cloves and add to pot.

Bring to a boil and then simmer, covered, until vegetables are tender. Remove the bouquet garni before puréeing the soup. I favor an immersion blender over a food processor for this, because I like just of bit of texture in the soup.

Return soup to pot, add salt and pepper to taste and stir in the lemon juice.

Garnish with chopped Italian parsley and serve with a dollop of good plain yogurt.

Serves 6.

VEGAN, GLUTEN-FREE

THIS WARMING, SUBTLE SOUP, ADAPTED FROM *THE VOLUPTUOUS VEGAN* USES AN ENTIRE HEAD OF GARLIC, BUT I KNOW FROM MANY TASTE TESTS THAT NO ONE WILL GUESS. THE TRICK IS THE ROASTING. DEPENDING ON THE STOCK AND CONDIMENTS, IT CAN BE MEAT-BASED, VEGETARIAN, OR VEGAN.

celeriac soup

4 medium celeriacs

2-1/2 cups veal, chicken, or vegetable stock

salt and white pepper

1/2 cup whipping cream (optional)

Peel celeriacs and cut into small pieces. Hold the cut pieces in acidulated water. Drain celeriac and put in a saucepan with stock to cover, about 2 cups. Simmer until soft, about 30 minutes. Remove from heat, purée, and return to pan. Add salt and freshly ground white pepper to taste. Thin if desired with more stock or whipping cream.

Serves 4.

THIS SOUP IS FROM BRUCE NAFTALY, CO-PROPRIETOR OF LE GOURMAND IN SEATTLE. IN THE WORDS OF ITS CREATOR, "IT SOUNDS RATHER HOMELY, BUT IT'S WONDERFUL." JERUSALEM ARTICHOKES CAN BE SUBSTITUTED FOR THE CELERIAC.

fish soup from fujian

1/2 pound firm fish fillet

1-1/2 tablespoons light soy sauce

1/4 teaspoon red pepper flakes

1 teaspoon cornstarch

1/2 teaspoon salt

1 tablespoon sesame oil

1 quart chicken stock

2 big slices fresh ginger

2 cups thinly sliced bok choy

⇥ cook's note

The rich, strong tamari soy sauce I usually favor is too strong here. If you must use it, cut back to 1 tablespoon

Slice fish into 1/4-inch strips. Blend soy sauce, red pepper flakes, cornstarch, salt, and sesame oil. Toss with fish strips and let stand 15 minutes.

Bring stock to a boil. Add fresh ginger and bok choy. Lower heat to simmer for 5 minutes. Gently add fish mixture and stir carefully. Cover and simmer 5 minutes.

Serves 4.

THIS IS SO EASY. YOU CAN WALK IN THE DOOR AT 7 AND HAVE IT ON THE TABLE AT 7:20. IT'S GOOD WITH CHINESE CABBAGE AS WELL AS BOK CHOY, AND I'VE EVEN MADE IT WITH ROMAINE IN A PINCH.

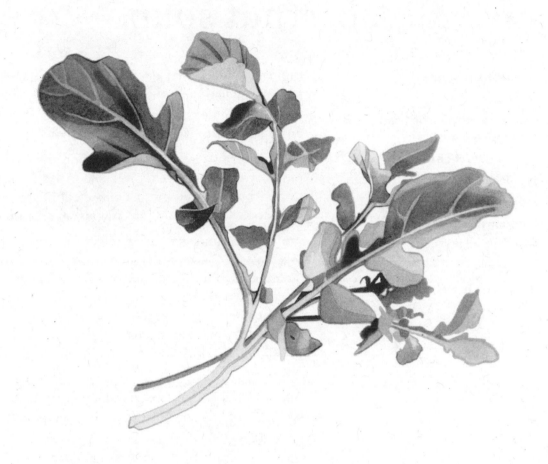

arugula

· · · · · · · · · · · · · · · · · · · ·

chestnut soup

1 pound fresh chestnuts

1/4 cup butter

6 to 8 shallots, minced, or 1 small yellow onion, chopped

1/2 cup celeriac, chopped fine

2 cups chicken stock

salt and white pepper

1/8 teaspoon nutmeg

1 cup half-and-half

chopped parsley

pickled ginger (available in Asian markets)

Cut a slash on the flat side of each chestnut shell. Simmer in water to cover until they are quite soft, about 15 minutes. Remove nuts from water, shell, and remove brown skins with a sharp knife.

Heat butter in a large saucepan. Sauté shallots or onion over medium heat until golden. Add chestnuts. Cook about a minute to coat outside of nuts and seal in flavors. Stir constantly to keep from burning.

Add celeriac and stir well. Add chicken stock. Bring to a boil, then cover and reduce heat. Simmer 20 to 30 minutes or until chestnuts are very tender. Strain chestnuts, shallot or onion, and celeriac from stock. Return stock to pan. Purée chestnuts and vegetables and return them to saucepan, stirring well. Bring mixture to a boil. Season with salt, white pepper, and nutmeg.

Add half-and-half. Reheat but do not boil. Ladle into bowls. Garnish each bowl with chopped parsley and a slice of pickled ginger.

Serves 4 to 6.

THIS RECIPE IS FROM JOHN DOERPER, WHOSE BOOKS AND MAGAZINE COLUMNS
SING THE PRAISES AND CHASTISE THE SHORTCOMINGS OF NORTHWEST KITCHENS.
THE GINGER SAVES THE DISH FROM OVERPOWERING RICHNESS. DOERPER USES WHIPPING
CREAM AND TOPS EACH SERVING WITH A SPOONFUL OF SALMON CAVIAR.
I CAN'T HANDLE THAT MUCH HIGH LIVING.

spicy chestnut soup

2 pounds fresh chestnuts or 1 pound canned unsweetened chestnut purée

1 quart vegetable stock

1 cup finely grated carrot or salsify

2 tablespoons butter

2 tablespoons flour

1/2 cup red wine

1/4 teaspoon nutmeg

1/4 teaspoon cayenne

salt and pepper

paprika

finely chopped parsley

If chestnuts are fresh, cut a slash on the flat side of each shell. Simmer in water to cover for 15 minutes or roast in the oven 15 to 20 minutes at 375°F. Peel chestnuts and purée, adding a bit of the vegetable stock if necessary. Add purée and grated carrot or salsify to remaining stock and simmer slowly for about 30 minutes.

Melt butter in another pot. Sprinkle in flour and cook, stirring, until roux begins to color. Add hot soup slowly to roux, whisking to keep it well blended. Add wine, nutmeg, cayenne, salt, and pepper, and simmer another 10 minutes over very low heat, stirring often.

Sprinkle a little paprika and parsley over each serving.

Serves 6.

VEGETARIAN

THIS IS A REAL DEPARTURE FROM THE MILD, CREAMY SOUPS USUALLY MADE WITH CHESTNUTS. IT HAS A FULL, DARK TASTE, ENLIVENED WITH CAYENNE.

italian greens and rice soup

1 pound escarole or chicory

3 tablespoons olive oil

2 teaspoons finely chopped garlic

1 small onion, chopped

salt

5 cups chicken broth

1/2 cup long-grain rice

black pepper

Parmesan cheese

Separate all the leaves of the escarole or chicory. Soak briefly in basin of water, drain, and cut crosswise into pieces about 1 inch wide.

Heat olive oil in heavy soup kettle and sauté garlic and onion until onion is pale gold, about 3 minutes. Add escarole or chicory, sprinkle lightly with salt, and cook 3 minutes more. Add 1 cup of broth, cover, and cook over low heat until escarole is quite tender, 10 to 15 minutes.

Add rest of broth and bring to boil. Add rice, cover, and simmer about 12 minutes or until rice is tender but firm to the bite. Taste and correct seasonings, add several grinds of black pepper.

Sprinkle with Parmesan cheese just before serving.

Serves 4.

THE SLIGHT BITTERNESS OF COOKED ESCAROLE OR CHICORY IS JUST RIGHT
WITH THE MILD FLAVORS OF CHICKEN AND RICE. A GREAT, SIMPLE SOUP.

fennel and shallot soup

1 tablespoon butter

1 cup shallots, peeled and chopped

2 cups chicken stock

2 pounds fennel (about 2 large bulbs), trimmed, cored and sliced

1 tablespoon fennel seeds

1/2 cup half-and-half

1/2 cup sour cream

salt and pepper

1/4 cup minced fennel tops

2 tablespoons grated Parmesan cheese (optional)

Melt butter in large, heavy saucepan over low heat. Add shallots and cook, stirring often, about 10 minutes or until they begin to soften. Add stock, fennel bulbs, and fennel seeds. Simmer until fennel is very tender, about 30 minutes, stirring occasionally. (Soup can be made ahead up to this point and refrigerated for a day or two.)

Press soup through a sieve, return to saucepan, and bring to a simmer. Whisk in half-and-half and sour cream. Season with salt and pepper. Add fennel tops. Ladle soup into bowls. Garnish with Parmesan cheese if desired.

Serves 4.

SHALLOTS ARE A VEGETABLE LUXURY THAT YOU CAN INDULGE IN QUANTITY IF YOU HAVE ANY GARDEN SPACE AT ALL. THE PINKISH-BROWN BULBS ARE EASY TO GROWN AND EXTREMELY HARDY, AND FOLIAGE IS DECORATIVE (OR AT LEAST UNOBTRUSIVE) ENOUGH TO COMBINE WITH ORNAMENTALS. AT MY OLD HOUSE, I GREW SHALLOTS, COLUMBINE, EGGPLANT AND LARKSPUR IN A SUNNY STRIP UNDER A WINDOW. IT WAS GORGEOUS. NOW THEY HANG OUT WITH THE MARJORAM IN AN HERB POT ON THE DECK. LITTLE YELLOW MULTIPLIER ONIONS ARE SOMETIMES MARKETED AS SHALLOTS IN GARDEN STORES. SHALLOTS TASTE BETTER.

gardeners green soup

3 tablespoons butter

half a medium onion, chopped

2 medium potatoes, peeled and diced

1 quart chicken stock

salt and pepper

2 cups sorrel leaves or a combination
of mild greens

2 tablespoons dry sherry

1/2 cup cream

fresh nutmeg

chopped parsley

chopped chives

Melt butter in a heavy saucepan and cook onion until soft but not brown. Add potatoes and cover with stock. Season with salt and pepper and simmer until potatoes are tender, about 15 minutes.

Pour a cup of soup and a handful of greens into the blender or food processor and purée at high speed. Repeat until all the soup and greens are blended. The mixture should be a nice, fresh green.

Return mixture to saucepan, add sherry, and reheat. Add a little more stock or water if soup is very thick. Stir in cream, heat, and correct seasoning. Add several grinds of fresh nutmeg.

Serve hot, garnished with parsley and chives.

Serves 6.

VERSIONS OF THIS SOUP APPEAR IN A NUMBER OF BOOKS, CREDITED TO MEALTIME INSPIRATIONS OF GARDENERS ON BOTH SIDES OF THE ATLANTIC. IT ALSO BEARS A RESEMBLANCE TO THE 18TH-CENTURY RECIPE FOR POTAGE PARMENTIER. SOME RECIPES CALL FOR A COMBINATION OF SPINACH AND SORREL, OR YOU COULD REPLACE THE SORREL WITH WATERCRESS OR ARUGULA. BECAUSE THE GREENS ARE BARELY COOKED, THIS IS NOT THE PLACE FOR TOUGH CUSTOMERS LIKE COLLARDS AND CHARD.

innisfree jerusalem artichoke and fennel soup

4 tablespoons butter or oil

2 leeks, sliced lengthwise and cut into half-rounds

3 celery stalks, diced

1 small fennel bulb, diced

1 teaspoon chopped parsley

1 teaspoon fresh or dried dill weed

salt and pepper

2 to 3 pounds Jerusalem artichokes, scrubbed and coarsely chopped

2 large potatoes, scrubbed and diced

2 quarts chicken or vegetable stock

1 cup half-and-half or nonfat yogurt

fennel leaves, for garnish

Melt butter or oil in medium soup pot. Add leeks, celery, and fennel and sauté until vegetables are just beginning to soften, 3 or 4 minutes. Add parsley, dill, salt, and pepper. Stir. Add Jerusalem artichokes, potatoes, and stock and bring to a simmer. Cook until artichokes are just tender, 15 to 20 minutes. Remove from heat. Purée about two-thirds of soup and return to pot. Add half-and-half or yogurt, stir, and heat through. Serve in heated bowls, garnished with fennel.

Serves 4 to 6.

MY FRIENDS FRED AND LYNN BERMAN SPECIALIZE IN FRESH SEASONAL FOOD, AND FRESH PASTA, AND AMAZING DESSERTS, AT THEIR BELLINGHAM, WASHINGTON, RESTAURANT, PASTAZZA. FARMERS AS WELL AS COOKS, THEY REALLY KNOW HOW TO BLEND THE FLAVORS THAT ARE READY TO HARVEST TOGETHER. THE FENNEL IS JUST ENOUGH TO PROVIDE INTRIGUE WITHOUT DOMINATING PLAINER TASTES. THE NAME COMES FROM THEIR FIRST RESTAURANT IN THE MOUNT BAKER FOOTHILLS.

jerusalem artichoke soup provençale

2 pounds Jerusalem artichokes, scrubbed and diced

6 cups water

salt

1 cup milk

2 tablespoons olive oil

1/2 cup drained canned tomatoes

1 clove garlic, crushed

1 tablespoon chopped parsley

2 tablespoons chopped ham or cooked bacon (optional)

Bring salted water to boil, add artichokes, lower heat, and cook until tender. Purée and return to heat. Add milk gradually and heat slowly. Heat olive oil in a small skillet; add tomatoes, garlic, parsley, and ham or bacon (if used). Cook briefly, no more than 2 minutes, and then pour mixture into artichoke purée. Heat to just below boiling and serve hot.

Serves 6.

(POTAGE DE TOPINAMBOURS À LA PROVENÇALE)

JERUSALEM ARTICHOKES GO WELL WITH A LITTLE HAM OR BACON. THE FLAVOR IS SIMILAR TO THAT OF A TRADITIONAL HAM AND BEAN SOUP, BUT THIS SOUP IS MUCH LIGHTER. IT'S ALSO ONE OF THE FASTEST SOUPS BECAUSE JERUSALEM ARTICHOKES COOK VERY QUICKLY.

jerusalem artichoke and sweet potato soup

2 tablespoons olive oil

3 shallots or 1/2 cup chopped onions

1 pound Jerusalem artichokes, scrubbed and sliced

1 large sweet potato, peeled and sliced

3 cups stock

1 bay leaf

1/2 cup milk or cream

salt and pepper

1 teaspoon lemon juice

1 tablespoon chopped Italian parsley

1/2 teaspoon paprika

Heat the olive oil in a heavy saucepan. Add the shallots or onions and sauté until translucent. Add the Jerusalem artichoke, sweet potato, stock and bay leaf and simmer until the roots are soft, about 30 minutes.

Remove from heat, remove bay leaf, and purée the mixture. Return mixture to saucepan, mix in milk or cream as desired, and heat gently. Don't let it boil.

Stir in salt, pepper, and lemon juice to taste. Sprinkle with parsley and paprika before serving. Pass around a bowl of good olive oil to drizzle on top.

Serves 4.

COMFORT FOOD OF A HIGH ORDER. YOU COULD LEAVE OUT THE MILK ENTIRELY; IT'S A MATTER OF PREFERRED TASTE AND TEXTURE. BOTH THE JERUSALEM ARTICHOKE AND THE SWEET POTATO MAKE A VERY SMOOTH PURÉE.

caldo verde

3 tablespoons olive oil

1 or more cloves garlic

1 medium leek with 2 inches green, chopped

2 medium potatoes, scrubbed and diced

1 linguiça, chorizo or other spicy sausage, sliced

5 cups chicken or vegetable stock

1 pound kale or collards (one large bunch), shredded, with tough ribs removed

salt and pepper

Heat olive oil in soup kettle, add garlic and leek, and sauté gently until leek becomes transparent. Add potatoes, sausage, and stock. Bring to boil and simmer until potatoes are tender, about 10 minutes. Add shredded kale or collards and cook another 5 to 10 minutes, depending on toughness of kale. Add salt and pepper to taste and serve hot.

Drizzle another tablespoon of good olive oil on top before serving.

Serves 6.

THIS IS PORTUGAL'S BEST-KNOWN SOUP, AND IT ALSO MARKS ONE OF THE EARLY USES OF THE POTATO IN EUROPEAN COOKING. IT IS AN EPITOME OF TRADITIONAL MEDITERRANEAN HOMESTEAD COOKING; FOR MOST FAMILIES, EVERY INGREDIENT WAS PRODUCED AT HOME. THE SIMPLE VEGETABLE BACKDROP SHOWED OFF THE FLAVORINGS OF REGIONAL SAUSAGES. WHEN TIMES WERE HARD AND THE HOUSEHOLD SAUSAGE SUPPLY WAS GONE, FAMILIES POURED THE MEATLESS SOUP OVER CRUSTY SLICES OF BREAD. VEGETARIANS CAN USE THE SAME METHOD TODAY, INCREASING THE GARLIC TO COMPENSATE FOR THE MISSING SAUSAGE SPICES. I HAVE ALSO SEEN VERSIONS WITH TEMPEH SUBSTITUTING FOR THE MEAT. THE KALE IS COOKED ONLY BRIEFLY, SO BE SURE AND SHRED IT INTO SMALL STRIPS. THE TUSCAN (AKA BLACK PALM) KALE IS A GOOD CHOICE HERE. IT'S PART-CABBAGE PEDIGREE GIVES THE LEAVES A BIT OF EXTRA HEFT, AND MAKES IT ESPECIALLY GOOD IN SOUPS AND STEWS. OTHER KALES, WINTER CABBAGE, OR COLLARDS, ALSO WORK WELL. IT'S A FINE USE FOR GREENS THAT ARE A BIT WEATHER-BEATEN BUT STILL FLAVORFUL. SOME RECIPES CALL FOR PURÉEING THE POTATOES. I PREFER THEM SIMPLY DICED, BUT IT'S A MATTER OF TASTE.

soupe bonne femme

2 large or 4 medium leeks

3 tablespoons butter

1/2 cup coarsely chopped onion

2 medium potatoes, diced

salt

3 cups boiling water or chicken stock

2 cups hot milk

chopped parsley or chives

Cut leeks in half lengthwise and then slice crosswise into 1/2-inch pieces. Wash and dry.

Melt 2 tablespoons of butter in a heavy saucepan, add leeks and onion, and cook over low heat, covered, until translucent, about 5 minutes. Stir frequently and don't let them brown. Add potatoes, salt, and boiling water. Bring to boil, cover, and simmer 25 minutes.

Add hot milk and remaining butter and serve hot, sprinkled with parsley or chives.

Serves 4.

LOUIS DIAT, THE RITZ-CARLTON CHEF AND CREATOR OF VICHYSSOISE, SAID HIS FAMILY USED TO HAVE THIS HOT POTATO-LEEK SOUP FOR BREAKFAST. IF YOU WANT TO FOLLOW HIS EXAMPLE, YOU COULD DO THE SIMMERING THE NIGHT BEFORE AND ADD THE HOT MILK IN THE MORNING. (DIAT IS ALSO SUPPOSED TO HAVE SAID THAT THERE ARE FIVE ELEMENTS—EARTH, AIR, FIRE, WATER, AND GARLIC—WHICH MAKES ME LIKE HIM EVEN MORE, THOUGH GARLIC IS NOT A FEATURE OF THIS SOOTHING BLEND.) VICHYSSOISE-LOVING GARDENERS CAN ENSURE A SUMMER SUPPLY BY MAKING POTATO-LEEK PURÉE IN QUANTITY, JUST BEFORE THEIR LEEKS BOLT TO SEED. IT FREEZES WELL. WHEN HOT WEATHER COMES, JUST THAW THE PURÉE AND COMPLETE YOUR FAVORITE RECIPE.

squash and leek soup

3 large leeks, white parts only, chopped

2 pounds winter squash, peeled and cubed

2 tablespoons olive oil

3 cups chicken or vegetable stock

1/2 cup milk or cream

salt and pepper

nutmeg

Heat the olive oil in a heavy saucepan. Add the leeks and sauté gently 3 or 4 minutes until they soften. Don't let them brown. Add the cubed squash, stir to coat with oil, and sauté another minute or two. Add stock, bring to boil, and then simmer, covered, until squash is soft.

Purée mixture. Then add the milk or cream and simmer 5 minutes to blend flavors. Stir in salt and pepper to taste, sprinkle with grated nutmeg, and serve hot.

Serves 4.

LARRY GONICK IS BEST KNOWN FOR HIS RECENTLY COMPLETED THIRTY-YEAR PROJECT, THE *CARTOON HISTORY OF THE UNIVERSE*, WHICH COVERS SCIENCE, HISTORY, AND GOOFY JOKES FROM THE BIG BANG TO 2008. HE IS ALSO AN OLD FRIEND AND A TERRIFIC COOK WHO HAS PUBLISHED A SERIES OF CARTOON RECIPES. THIS CHEERY GOLDEN VARIATION ON SOUPE BONNE FEMME IS ONE EXAMPLE. THE BETTER FLAVORED THE SQUASH, THE BETTER THE SOUP. USE A KABOCHA IF YOU HAVE ONE.

mushroom ciorba

1/2 ounce dried porcini mushrooms

3 cups coarsely chopped fresh mushrooms

2 tablespoons butter

1 leek, white part only, chopped fine

1 medium onion, chopped fine

2 cups vegetable or beef broth

1 cup sauerkraut juice

salt and pepper

1/2 cup sour cream or whole-milk yogurt

chopped chives or green onion for garnish

Soak the dried mushrooms, covered, in about 1/3 cup warm water for an hour.

While dried mushrooms are soaking, sauté the leek and onion in the butter until they start to soften. Add fresh mushrooms and cook, stirring occasionally, until they are soft and most of the liquid has evaporated.

Add broth, sauerkraut juice, salt and pepper. Simmer, uncovered, for about 20 minutes.

Drain the soaked dried mushrooms and reserve the liquid. Strain it to remove any pieces of dirt. Chop the mushrooms and add them to the soup with their strained liquid.

Remove soup from heat, stir in sour cream and lemon juice, and reheat to a simmer. Do not let it boil. Sprinkle with green onions or chives and serve.

Serves 4 to 6.

A REAL BALKAN AMALGAM OF FLAVORS, THIS ROMANIAN SOUP GETS A THREE-WAY ADDITION OF SATISFYING SOURNESS FROM SAUERKRAUT, LEMON JUICE, AND SOUR CREAM. IT'S IMPORTANT TO USE SOME GOOD DRIED MUSHROOMS RATHER THAN SUPERMARKET BUTTONS. I FAVOR BOLETES (KNOWN IN ITALY AS *PORCINI* AND IN EASTERN EUROPE AS *ČEP*). YOU NEED A BIT OF THEIR STRONGER FLAVOR TO STAND UP TO THE KRAUT. THIS VERSION IS ADAPTED FROM *CROSSROADS COOKING*. TRADITIONALLY, IT HAS AN EGG MIXED IN, SIMILAR TO GREEK AVGOLEMONO, BUT I LIKE IT FINE WITHOUT.

mushroom soup

2 tablespoons butter

2 tablespoons oil

1 clove garlic, minced

1 to 2 pounds fresh mushrooms,
quartered if small, sliced if large

salt and pepper

1/4 cup dry sherry

1/2 teaspoon dried basil

1/2 cup chopped green onions or chives

2 tablespoons chopped parsley

6 cups chicken stock

freshly grated nutmeg

Heat butter and oil in a large saucepan. Add garlic and cook very gently for a few minutes. Don't let garlic brown. Add mushrooms, stir thoroughly, and sprinkle with salt and pepper. Cook uncovered over low heat for 15 to 20 minutes, stirring often, until liquid released by mushrooms has almost evaporated. Add sherry, basil, green onions or chives, and parsley and cook another 5 minutes. Add chicken stock, bring to a boil, and simmer 10 minutes. Remove 3 cups of the soup and purée. Return to saucepan and heat through. Serve hot with a little grated nutmeg.

Mom sometimes darkened the stock by cooking it with an onion peel. It gives a nice rich color. Don't forget to fish it out before you assemble the soup.

Serves 4 to 6.

MY MOTHER MADE THE BEST MUSHROOM SOUP IN THE WORLD. THIS IS MY BEST ATTEMPT TO QUANTIFY WHAT SHE DID BY INTUITION AND IMPROVISATION. THE ORIGINAL RECIPE, LONG LOST, CAME FROM HER FRIEND MYRTLE JAMES. THE SOUP CONTAINS NO MILK OR CREAM, SO THE MUSHROOM FLAVOR IS INTENSIFIED. IF YOU ARE A MUSHROOM GATHERER, THIS IS A GREAT SHOWCASE FOR YOUR FAVORITE FLAVORS.

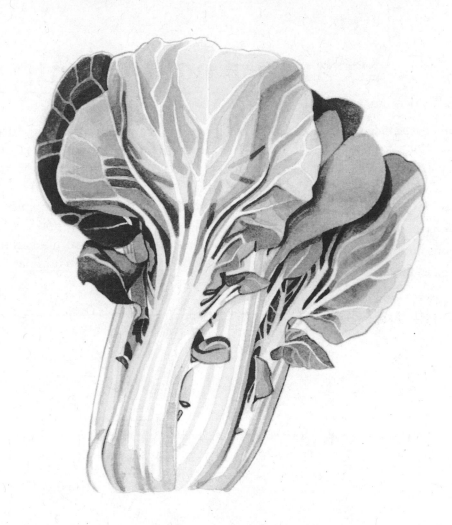

bok choy

cream of nettle soup

4 cups young nettle leaves (*see p. 26 for gathering and handling tips*)

2 cups chicken or vegetable stock

2 cups milk (soy milk is fine, though I wouldn't use low-fat)

2 tablespoons grated onion

2 tablespoons butter or canola oil

2 tablespoons flour

salt and pepper to taste

grated Parmesan cheese (optional)

Wash nettles and steam until soft in the water that clings to them. Purée with their liquid, adding some stock by the tablespoon if necessary. Melt butter in a medium saucepan, add onion, and cook until soft. Add flour and cook, stirring constantly, until color starts to turn. Add stock, salt, pepper, and nettle purée and heat to boiling. Lower heat and simmer 10 minutes. Add milk or cream and heat gently. Sprinkle each serving with Parmesan to taste.

Serves 4.

REVENGE IS ONE MOTIVE FOR EATING NETTLES, BUT THERE ARE OTHERS. THE PROLIFIC STINGING PLANT IS ONE OF THE EARLIEST GREENS UP IN THE SPRING; IT'S HIGH IN VITAMINS C AND K AND MINERALS, ESPECIALLY CALCIUM. NETTLE DISHES, ESPECIALLY SOUPS, ARE TRADITIONAL IN FRENCH, SCOTTISH, AND WELSH COOKING. SOURCES OFTEN SAY IT TASTES LIKE SPINACH, BUT TO ME IT LACKS THAT BIT OF SWEETNESS THAT MAKES GOOD GARDEN SPINACH SO WONDERFUL. AND UNLIKE SPINACH, IT IS CERTAINLY NOT BEST RAW. USE GLOVES FOR ALL NETTLE-RELATED TASKS UNTIL IT IS THOROUGHLY COOKED (AT LEAST 10 MINUTES), WHICH REMOVES THE ITCHY STING. THE STRONG, WILD FLAVOR HOLDS UP ESPECIALLY WELL WHEN LIGHTENED WITH A SPLASH OF GOOD BALSAMIC VINEGAR OR NESTLED INTO AN OMELET OR IN A CREAMY SOUP LIKE THIS ONE.

oyster parsnip stew

1/4 pound (4 strips), lean bacon, diced

1 medium onion, chopped

4 cups total more or less equal quantities of scrubbed, diced parsnips and potatoes

2 cups boiling water

1 small jar oysters, with their liquid

3 cups milk, scalded (I use 2 percent; you won't miss the extra cream here)

1-1/2 cups chopped spinach

salt and pepper

Cook bacon slowly in a heavy saucepan or flameproof casserole until it begins to crisp. Add the chopped onion and sauté until golden. I use very lean Hempler's bacon and sometimes have to add a bit of olive oil to keep the onions from burning. Add parsnips and potatoes, stirring to coat them well. Cook, stirring, about 5 minutes over medium heat.

Drain the oyster liquid into a measuring cup and add enough of the boiling water to make 2 cups. Add liquid to vegetable mixture, lower heat to simmer, and cook, covered, until roots are tender, about 20 minutes. Remove a cup or two of the vegetable mixture (it depends on how thick you like your stew), blend or purée, and return to the pot.

Add milk, spinach, and oysters and simmer another 5 minutes. Season to taste with salt and pepper.

Serves 6.

GLUTEN-FREE

I LOVE OYSTER STEW, AND IT TAKES A LOT TO MOVE ME FROM THE PURIST BASICS—LOTS OF OYSTERS, MILK, A SMIDGEON OF HAM OR BACON, AND A POTATO OR TWO. BUT I'M CRAZY ABOUT THIS VERSION, AND RIGHT NOW IT IS MY FAVORITE THING TO DO WITH PARSNIPS. THE SPINACH IS PRETTY, AND IT TURNS OUT TO BE THE PERFECT BRIDGE BETWEEN SWEET PARSNIP AND MINERAL OYSTER FLAVORS. PURÉEING SOME OF THE VEGETABLES IN PLACE OF THE USUAL ROUX LIGHTENS THE DISH, HIGHLIGHTS THE OTHER FLAVORS (AND MAKES THE DISH GLUTEN-FREE). IF YOU HAVE AFFORDABLE FRESH OYSTERS, BY ALL MEANS USE THEM.

two-pumpkin soup

2 tablespoons rendered goose fat, home-rendered lard, butter, or olive oil

1 medium leek, white part only, chopped

1 medium onion, chopped

3/4 cup pie pumpkin, peeled and diced

3/4 cup Hokkaido squash, peeled and diced

1 teaspoon ground juniper berries

2 cups white stock, made with veal, chicken, or vegetables

1/8 teaspoon white pepper

salt to taste

Heat fat or oil in a saucepan. Add leek and onion and sauté until soft. Add pumpkin, squash, and juniper berries and cook gently, stirring occasionally, for about 10 minutes. Add stock and simmer for about 30 minutes or until pumpkin and squash are soft. Remove from heat, purée, and return to pan. Thin as needed with more stock. Add pepper and salt to taste.

Serves 4.

Note to foragers: Juniper trees are common, but do not try gathering your own juniper berries unless you are an expert. Juniper berries are not really berries but a variant of conifer cones, and as such tend to be unpleasantly resinous. Only a few varieties are mild enough to keep your soup from tasting like retsina. Even if you *want* your soup to taste like retsina, the wrong berries also can cause digestive upsets.

A lot of pumpkin soups feature sweet spices and cream, and in truth they rather resemble pumpkin pie filling. I prefer savory spices with pumpkins and squash, such as this soup from Le Gourmand in Seattle, which is flavored with juniper berries. Bruce Naftaly makes it with pie pumpkin and Japanese Hokkaido squash. Feel free to substitute your own favorites. Bruce also sautés the vegetables in goose fat, but good results can be obtained with other fats and oils.

root vegetable and leek soup with gouda cheese

2 tablespoons butter

1 small onion, chopped

3 leeks, white and pale green parts, washed well and chopped fine

3 cups strong chicken stock

1 salsify root (or small amount of turnip or parsnip), peeled and grated

6 medium potatoes, peeled and chopped

salt and pepper

1 carrot, grated

2 cups milk

1 cup shredded Gouda cheese

chives (optional)

carrot rounds, cut into stars (optional)

Melt butter in large saucepan or soup pot. Add onion, leeks, and a little salt and sauté over medium heat, stirring, until soft, about 15 minutes. Don't rush this part—proper slow cooking brings out a certain natural sweetness.

Add chicken stock and salsify and heat to simmering. Add potatoes. Cover without stirring (you want the potatoes to stay on top) and cook until potatoes are tender, about 25 minutes. Lift out potatoes with a slotted spoon, purée, and return to soup. Add a little salt and a generous amount of pepper. Bring soup to a boil, add carrots, and stir in milk. Bring just to boiling, add cheese, adjust seasoning, and heat through. Do not boil again.

Serve in shallow bowls, sprinkled with chives and a few floated carrot stars, if used.

Serves 6 as a soup course or 3 as a main course.

THIS RUSTIC SOUP IS A PERFECT MARRIAGE OF FORM AND CONTENT. IT USES PLAIN WINTER INGREDIENTS TO PROVIDE THE COMFORT AND UPLIFT WE NEED ON GRAY DAYS. THE RECIPE IS FROM RON ZIMMERMAN, CHEF AT THE HERBFARM RESTAURANT IN THE CASCADE FOOTHILLS EAST OF SEATTLE. ZIMMERMAN USES YAKIMA VALLEY GOUDA. I LIKE PLEASANT VALLEY GOUDA, WHICH IS MADE NEAR MY HOME IN WHATCOM COUNTY. THE POINT IN THIS RECIPE IS NOT TO WORRY ABOUT BRAND NAMES BUT TO PAY THE PRICE FOR A GOOD-QUALITY CHEESE. IF YOUR EXPERIENCE WITH GOUDA IS LIMITED TO THOSE RUBBERY LITTLE HOCKEY PUCKS THAT GET PASSED AROUND AT CHRISTMASTIME, YOU'LL BE AMAZED AT HOW GOOD IT CAN BE.

spinach soup
with grain dumplings

4 tablespoons butter or olive oil

2 cups minced onion

2 quarts beef or vegetable stock

1-1/2 cups rolled oats

1/2 cup bulgur

1 teaspoon salt

1/4 teaspoon pepper

1/2 cup warm water

2 tablespoons tomato paste

1 tablespoon fresh lemon juice

1 pound fresh spinach (1 big bunch), chopped fine

Melt butter or oil in large soup kettle and sauté onion until translucent. Add stock and bring to a boil. In a mixing bowl combine rolled oats, bulgur, salt, and pepper. Add warm water and mix with fingers until batter is stiff. It will be sticky. Form into balls no more than 1 inch in diameter and drop into hot soup. Cover and simmer 20 minutes. Mix together tomato paste and lemon juice and add to soup along with spinach. Cover and simmer 3 to 5 minutes. Serve hot.

Serves 6.

I'M VERY FOND OF THIS UNUSUAL SOUP, WHICH COMBINES A HEARTY DUMPLING WITH A FRESH VEGETABLE TASTE.

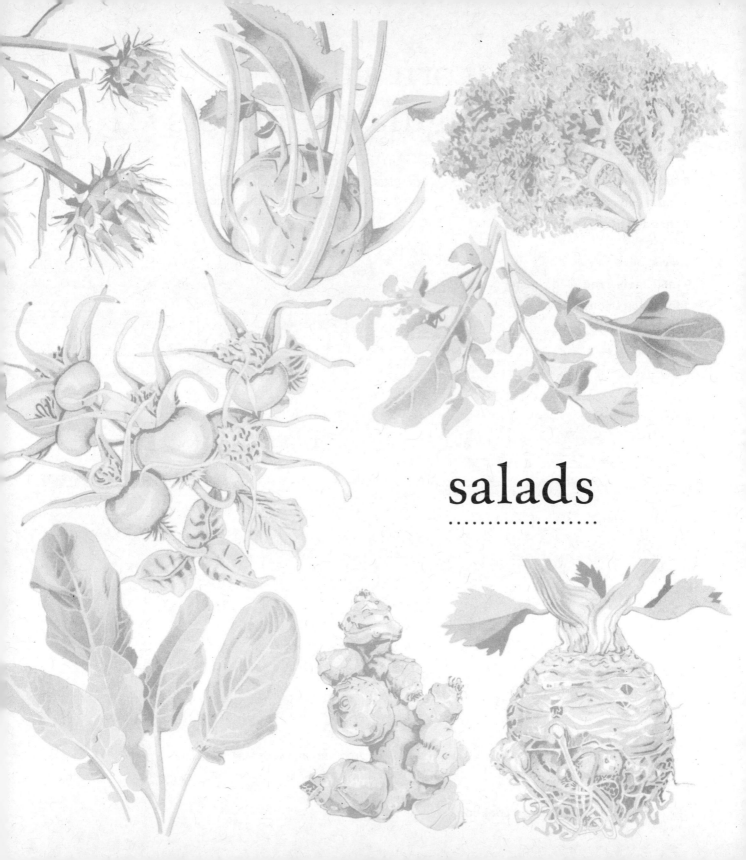

salads

corn salad
and arugula with beets

4 cups mixed corn salad and arugula

1 cup sliced cooked beets

2 chopped green onions or very small leeks

1/4 cup olive oil

3 tablespoons red wine vinegar

1 teaspoon Dijon mustard

salt and pepper

Wash greens, place in a bowl, and arrange beets and onions on top. Dress with oil, vinegar, mustard, and salt and pepper to taste.

Serves 4.

VEGAN

THIS IS A GARDENER'S SALAD, REPRINTED FROM THE NICHOLS GARDEN NURSERY CATALOG.
IT COMBINES TWO OF MY FAVORITE WINTER GREENS WITH BEETS.

beet salad
with garlic sauce

1 pound beets

3 tablespoons light-flavored olive oil

2 tablespoons red wine vinegar

1/2 small onion, sliced thin

1 cup skordalia (*see page 228*)

Simmer beets in 2 cups water until tender. Drain, reserving 2 tablespoons of the cooking liquid. When beets are cool enough to handle, peel, slice thin, and arrange in a serving bowl with onion slices.

Combine oil, vinegar, and cooking liquid, pour over vegetables, and mix well. Serve chilled, with skordalia.

Serves 4 to 6.

THIS IS A GOOD, SIMPLE SALAD, EVEN WITHOUT THE PUNGENT SKORDALIA.

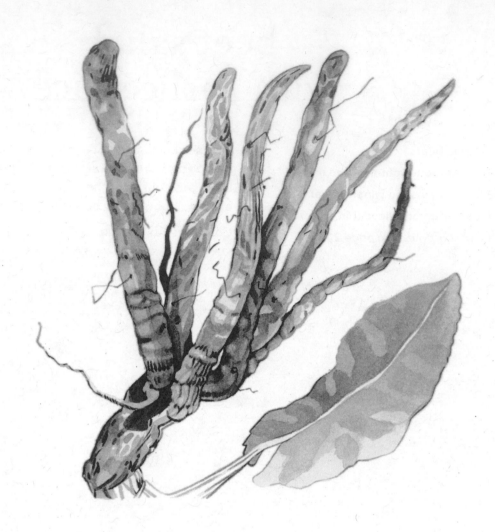

burdock

....

russian beet salad

1 pound beets

2 cloves garlic, minced

1/3 cup chopped walnuts

1/4 cup chopped prunes (soak prunes
for 20 minutes in hot water if they are
getting hard)

3 tablespoons mayonnaise

salt and pepper

Scrub beets and remove green tops. Bake at 375°F until
soft but not mushy, up to 2 hours, or in a microwave
oven for 15 minutes. When they are cool enough to
handle, slip off the skins and shred coarsely.

Combine beets with garlic, walnuts, and prunes.
Add mayonnaise and mix well. Season to taste
with salt and pepper and chill well before serving.

Serves 6.

VEGETARIAN

YOU DON'T HAVE TO ALREADY BE A BEET FAN TO LIKE THIS, ALTHOUGH YOU MUST
APPRECIATE GARLIC. THE DEEP RED BEETS AND NEON-PINK MAYONNAISE
MAKE A VIVID—NOT TO SAY ALARMING—COMBINATION.

brussels sprout salad

3 tablespoons fresh lemon juice, divided

1-1/2 cups sliced Jerusalem artichokes

1 large celeriac, peeled and sliced into bite-sized pieces (discard any corky center portion)

4 small leeks (white part only), chopped

1 pound fresh Brussels sprouts

3 tablespoons olive oil

1 tablespoon fresh grated lemon rind (optional)

salt and pepper

2 tablespoons chopped parsley

Combine 1 tablespoon of the lemon juice and 3 cups of water in a medium bowl. Add Jerusalem artichoke and celeriac slices and let stand, covered, in refrigerator until it's time to dress the salad.

Cook leeks in an inch of boiling, salted water until tender but not slimy, about 5 minutes. Drain, saving the water. Bring water back to a boil and steam Brussels sprouts only until crisp-tender, about 8 to 10 minutes.

Put leeks and Brussels sprouts in a serving bowl. Drain Jerusalem artichoke and celeriac well and add. Dress with olive oil, the remaining 2 tablespoons of lemon juice, and lemon rind (if used). Add salt and pepper to taste, mix, and check for seasoning.

Cover and let stand in refrigerator for an hour before serving. Garnish with chopped parsley.

Serves 4.

VEGAN, GLUTEN-FREE

USE SMALL, SWEET BRUSSELS SPROUTS. GARDENERS HAVE AN IMMENSE ADVANTAGE HERE, FOR ALTHOUGH BRUSSELS SPROUTS KEEP FAIRLY WELL, THEY HOLD THEIR PEAK OF FLAVOR ONLY BRIEFLY.

antibes coleslaw

1 small cabbage

1 garlic clove, crushed

6 tablespoons olive oil

2-1/2 tablespoons red or
white wine vinegar

3 or 4 anchovy fillets, packed in oil,
drained and minced

1 teaspoon Dijon mustard

salt and pepper

Wash cabbage, remove outer leaves, cut in half, and remove core. Slice thin. Combine remaining ingredients in small bowl, mix well, and blend with cabbage. Allow to stand for 10 minutes and serve.

Serves 6.

I DON'T MUCH LIKE MOST COLESLAW, BUT I LOVE THIS.

marinated cooked carrots

1/2 cup water
1/2 cup white wine vinegar
1/2 cup white wine or dry sherry
1/2 cup olive oil
1 tablespoon parsley, chopped
1 teaspoon fresh thyme, or pinch dried
1 teaspoon salt
1 clove garlic
pinch cayenne
1 pound carrots (about 6 medium), scrubbed and quartered
1/2 teaspoon smooth Dijon mustard

This is from the legendary British food writer Elizabeth David. Cooking the carrots briefly in the marinade gives them an intense flavor. They still should have a bit of crunch.

Bring to a boil all but the last two ingredients. Add carrots and cook, uncovered, at medium-high heat until they are barely tender. Drain carrots, reserving liquid. Arrange carrots in a serving bowl. Add mustard to liquid, mix well, and pour over carrots. Cool for at least an hour before serving.

Serves 6.

VEGAN

moroccan carrot salad

1 pound carrots (about 6 medium), scrubbed
2 shallots, chopped fine
2 to 3 tablespoons sugar
1/2 teaspoon salt
1/2 teaspoon ground cumin
pepper
dash cayenne
3 tablespoons lemon juice
1/2 cup finely minced parsley

Grate or julienne carrots. Add shallots and toss. Combine sugar, salt, and cumin and toss with carrots. Season with pepper and cayenne. Add lemon juice and toss again. Marinate for 1 hour. Sprinkle with parsley and serve at room temperature.

Serves 6.

VEGAN, GLUTEN-FREE

THE FIRST SUMMER CARROTS ARE SO SWEET AND CRISP AND BEAUTIFUL THAT IT WOULD BE COUNTERPRODUCTIVE TO DO ANYTHING MORE THAN SCRUB THEM. BY MID-WINTER, HOWEVER, MY GARDEN HOLDOVERS NEED SOME HELP TO LOOK AS GOOD AS THEY TASTE. THE QUALITY OF GROCERY CARROTS—ALWAYS VARIABLE—GETS MORE SO AS STORAGE TIME LENGTHENS. THIS IS THE TIME FOR MARINADES. HERE ARE TWO GOOD ONES.

celeriac and beet salad

2 medium beets

1 medium celeriac

1/3 cup olive oil

salt and pepper

juice of 2 lemons

Boil or bake beets; boiling is quicker, but roasting develops a richer flavor. Peel and julienne when cool enough to handle. Peel and slice celeriac and steam until just tender. Mix beets and celeriac. Make a dressing of olive oil, salt, pepper, and lemon juice. Pour over vegetables and chill before serving.

Serves 4 to 6.

VEGAN, GLUTEN-FREE

SERVED HOT, THIS ALSO MAKES A NICE SIDE DISH.

celeriac and shrimp
with mustard dressing

2 eggs

1 tablespoon Dijon mustard

2 teaspoons white wine vinegar

salt and pepper

3/4 cup light oil

3 small celeriacs, peeled and coarsely grated

1 tablespoon lemon juice

12 cooked deveined shrimp, cubed

minced chives or green onions

Mix eggs, mustard, vinegar, salt, and pepper in blender or food processor for about 30 seconds. Begin adding oil by drops and continue blending until mixture is thick and smooth. Taste and adjust seasonings if necessary.

Sprinkle celeriac with a little lemon juice. Add dressing. Toss with shrimp and chives or green onions until well blended. Chill 3 to 4 hours before serving.

Serves 6.

FRENCH COOKS WILL RECOGNIZE THIS AS A JAZZED-UP VERSION OF CELERIAC RÉMOULADE. HERE, THE CELERIAC IS GRATED RAW INSTEAD OF JULIENNED AND BLANCHED. SMALL ROOTS ARE BEST FOR THIS DISH. YOU COULD USE CRAB IN PLACE OF SHRIMP.

celeriac rémoulade

half a lemon

1 or 2 celeriac roots
(about 1 pound total)

2 tablespoons Dijon mustard

1 tablespoon red wine vinegar

salt and pepper

1/4 cup light oil

2 tablespoons chopped parsley

Cut lemon into two wedges. Squeeze one wedge into a medium bowl of water and the other into a saucepan with a quart of water. Bring water in saucepan to a boil. Meanwhile, peel celeriac and cut into julienne slices. There should be 3 to 4 cups. Keep unsliced pieces in the lemon water, and return the julienned slices to the lemon water as you prepare them. Drain slices and blanch briefly in the boiling water. Drain again and dry on a towel.

Whisk mustard, vinegar, salt, and pepper together in a large bowl. Add about 2 tablespoons of oil, beating energetically, and then add the rest in droplets, whisking all the while. Fold celeriac into the sauce and marinate for several hours. Garnish with chopped parsley just before serving.

Serves 4 to 6.

VEGAN

A CLASSIC OF FRENCH COOKING, SIMPLE AND SATISFYING.

endive and watercress salad

4 heads endive, cored and cut into bite-sized pieces

1 large bunch watercress (leaves and small stems only)

1 small clove garlic, cut lengthwise

4 tablespoons olive oil

salt and pepper

2 tablespoons red wine vinegar

Rub salad bowl with garlic. Combine endive, cress, and olive oil in salad bowl and toss. Add salt, pepper, and vinegar and toss again.

Serves 4.

VEGAN, GLUTEN-FREE

IF YOU GROW YOUR OWN ENDIVE, THIS HIGH-TICKET SALAD IS SUDDENLY AFFORDABLE. EVEN IF YOU DON'T, IT'S WORTH IT ONCE IN A WHILE.

fennel and apple salad

2 heads fennel, trimmed and chopped

4 medium apples, cored and chopped

2 tablespoons lemon juice

salt and pepper

1/4 cup sunflower seeds

3 tablespoons oil

2 teaspoons sugar

watercress (optional)

Put fennel and apples in a bowl, sprinkle with lemon juice, and mix. Add salt, pepper, and sunflower seeds and mix again. Dissolve sugar in oil, pour over salad, and mix. Garnish with watercress if you like.

Serves 6.

VEGAN, GLUTEN-FREE

IF YOU DON'T ALREADY LIKE FENNEL, THIS PROBABLY WON'T CHANGE YOUR MIND, BUT IF YOU DO, IT'S A NICE FRESH TASTE.

kohlrabi salad

4 small kohlrabi, peeled

salt

2 tablespoons soy sauce

1/2 teaspoon sugar

1 teaspoon hot pepper sauce

3 tablespoons toasted sesame oil

3 stalks celery, chopped, or 1 cup chopped celeriac

3 or 4 green onions, chopped

Grate kohlrabi, sprinkle with salt, and let stand for 30 minutes. Rinse and drain. Blend soy sauce, sugar, and hot pepper sauce. Gradually add sesame oil, whisking constantly. Add kohlrabi, celery or celeriac, and green onions, toss, and chill for at least 1 hour. Toss again before serving.

Serves 4.

VEGAN

LIKE ITS BROCCOLI COUSIN, KOHLRABI RESPONDS BEAUTIFULLY TO SOY SAUCE
AND SESAME FLAVORS. SMALL ONES ARE BEST FOR SALADS.

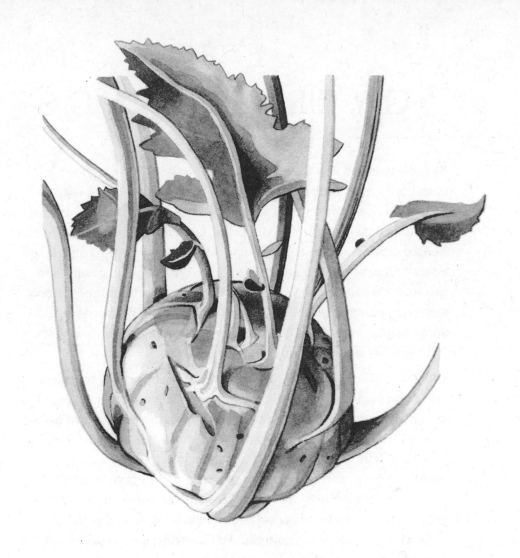

kohlrabi

· ·

GREEN SALADS

Flexibility is the key to winter green salads. If you go shopping with your heart set on a Caesar, you might come home with a brownish head of romaine when you could have had a perfectly nice spinach salad for half the price. Likewise, gardeners need to head outdoors with an open mind. Unless you garden on a large scale or live alone, you are unlikely to have enough of any one green in December or January. When it comes to combinations, anything you like goes. Like the gourmet salad mixtures sold at some farmers markets and groceries, your salads will vary with the weather and your fancy.

I prefer rather simple salads, and I try for contrasting textures and complementary flavors. Arugula and corn salad make a nice mix of spice and bland, and some chopped leeks or green onions give a little crunch. Arugula and mustard greens together would be overkill, unless you really like it hot and don't mind a coarse texture. Sorrel and spinach are an easy, pretty combination. The leaves are similar in shape and size, but the sorrel is a lighter green. I think most winter salads should be dressed with a fairly plain vinaigrette; more complicated dressings can clash with the many-flavored greens.

Keep in mind that almost everything harvested in mid-winter will taste stronger than the same plant in its tender spring growth. Also, even the toughest greens suffer some structural damage in freezing weather. They won't be as crisp as they were in October. Harvest and clean them very gently to avoid bruising.

tibetan salad

1 bunch fresh spinach

1 bunch watercress

1 teaspoon honey

2 cloves garlic, crushed

1/2 teaspoon red pepper flakes

salt

1/4 cup hot water

1 cup yogurt

1 tablespoon vegetable oil

1/4 teaspoon fenugreek seeds

Remove stems from greens and wash leaves gently and thoroughly. Drain well and chop coarsely. Put greens in a salad bowl. Mix honey, garlic, red pepper flakes, and salt to taste in a small cup and add hot water. Stir until honey is dissolved, add yogurt, and pour over salad. Mix gently. Heat oil in a small pan or skillet; add fenugreek seeds and sauté until they soften, about 2 or 3 minutes. Pour over salad.

Serves 4.

GLUTEN-FREE

TIBETANS MAKE THIS SALAD FROM BUCKWHEAT GREENS, ONE OF THE VERY FEW LEAFY VEGETABLES THAT CAN GROW IN THEIR EXTREME CLIMATE. GARDENERS WHO USE BUCKWHEAT AS A SUMMER COVER CROP CAN EXPERIENCE THE AUTHENTIC TASTE. BUCKWHEAT GREENS ARE HARD TO COME BY IN WINTER (THOUGH SPROUTING SEEDS ARE EASILY AVAILABLE; YOU COULD TRY THAT VARIATION), BUT MY FRIEND RINJING DORJE, CO-AUTHOR OF *FOOD IN TIBETAN LIFE*, WHENCE THIS RECIPE COMES, SAYS A COMBINATION OF SPINACH AND WATERCRESS MAKES A GOOD SUBSTITUTE. FENUGREEK SEEDS ARE AS HARD AS THE LITTLE ROCKS THEY RESEMBLE, BUT THEY SOFTEN WHEN COOKED. INCIDENTALLY, FENUGREEK IS EASY TO GROW IN NORTHWEST GARDENS, AND THE BITTER GREENS CAN BE USED WITH DISCRETION IN SALADS. RICHTERS HERB SPECIALISTS OUT OF GOODWOOD, ONTARIO, HAS SEED BY THE PACKET AND BY THE KILO. ONE EXAMPLE OF HOW FORMERLY ARCANE KNOWLEDGE IS NOW INSTANTLY ACCESSIBLE IS THAT YOU CAN NOW GOOGLE A FENUGREEK SPROUTING VIDEO ON YOUTUBE.

historic salad

8 hard-boiled eggs

1 head Boston lettuce or other Bibb-type lettuce

1 fennel bulb, sliced

4 medium beets, baked or boiled, peeled, and chopped fine

8 anchovy fillets (optional)

2 teaspoons chopped parsley

1 teaspoon chopped fresh chervil (optional)

1 teaspoon chopped fresh tarragon or 1/2 teaspoon dried

1 teaspoon chopped chives

1 teaspoon chopped capers

1/4 cup olive oil

3 tablespoons red wine vinegar

Peel and quarter eggs. Line a salad bowl with lettuce leaves. Arrange eggs on lettuce, add fennel slices, sprinkle with chopped beets, and crisscross anchovies (if used) over the top. Put herbs and capers in a jar with a lid, add olive oil and vinegar, close tightly, and shake until blended. Pour over salad just before serving.

Serves 8.

THIS UPDATED 17TH-CENTURY RECIPE IS FROM *COURT AND COUNTRY COOK*,
AN ENGLISH TRANSLATION OF AN EARLY FRENCH COOKBOOK. IT IS NOT FOR
THE FAINT OF PALATE, BUT IT'S GOOD. YOU COULD REDUCE OR OMIT
THE ANCHOVIES AND STILL HAVE PLENTY OF FLAVOR.

watercress raita

· ·

1 cup watercress leaves, chopped

2 cups plain yogurt

1 clove garlic, chopped

pinch of cayenne

Combine watercress, yogurt, and garlic in a blender, or reduce watercress and garlic to a paste with a mortar and pestle and then stir in yogurt. (The raita will be thinner if you use a blender.) Sprinkle with cayenne and refrigerate until time to serve.

Makes 2 cups.

VEGETARIAN, GLUTEN-FREE

radish raita

· ·

1 cup grated radish (red or daikon)

2 teaspoons salt

2 cups plain yogurt

1/8 teaspoon ground cumin

pinch of cayenne

Put grated radish in a bowl. Add salt and knead to squeeze out excess water. In another bowl, beat yogurt with a fork until smooth. Add radish and cumin and mix well. Sprinkle with cayenne and refrigerate until time to serve.

Makes 2 cups.

VEGETARIAN, GLUTEN-FREE

RAITAS ARE YOGURT-BASED ACCOMPANIMENTS TO INDIAN MEALS. THEY ARE SIMPLE TO MAKE AND PRETTY, AND THEY ADD IMMEASURABLY TO A CURRY OR PILAF. MOST FOLLOW THE SAME BASIC PATTERN, SO IT'S EASY TO INVENT YOUR OWN USING CARROTS, CABBAGE, BANANAS, OR WHATEVER ELSE SOUNDS TASTY. RAITAS DON'T KEEP WELL; CUT THE RECIPES IN HALF IF LEFTOVERS ARE A PROBLEM.

rutachoke salad

1/2 cup grated rutabaga

1/2 cup grated Jerusalem artichoke

2 green onions or small leeks, chopped

2 radishes, sliced thin

3 cups shredded romaine

DRESSING

3 tablespoons olive oil

1 tablespoon wine vinegar

salt and pepper

1/4 teaspoon dry mustard

1/4 teaspoon dried basil

⊰ cook's note

It is hard to determine a rutabaga's sweetness and texture from it's size or appearance. Small ones can be hot and woody; huge ones can be sweet and crisp. Try a bit raw before committing yourself to any particular root.

Combine vegetables in salad bowl and chill well. Combine dressing ingredients in a jar, shake, and chill. Dress and toss just before serving.

Serves 4.

VEGAN

YELLOW RUTABAGA AND COLORFUL RADISH PERK UP THIS ATTRACTIVE SALAD.

sprout salad

2 cups sprouts, rinsed (*see note below*)

1 medium carrot, grated

1 small turnip, peeled and grated

2 minced shallots or 2 tablespoons minced onion

1 cup sliced mushrooms (optional)

2 tablespoons soy sauce

2 teaspoons grated ginger

3 tablespoons oil

2 tablespoons rice wine vinegar

1 tablespoon toasted sesame seeds

toasted sesame oil

Mix together sprouts, carrot, turnip, shallots or onion, and mushrooms (if used). Combine soy sauce, ginger, oil, and rice wine vinegar and pour over salad. Sprinkle with sesame seeds and a few shakes of sesame oil.

Serves 4.

VEGAN

YOU NEED SPROUTS WITH SOME BODY HERE; ALFALFA SPROUTS ARE TOO TENDER. I FAVOR THE MIXED SPROUT PACKAGES YOU CAN BUY IN MANY SUPERMARKETS. OTHERWISE, USE SUNFLOWER OR MUNG BEAN SPROUTS. POWDERED GINGER WON'T WORK IN THIS RECIPE. IF YOU USE FRESH GINGER ONLY OCCASIONALLY, YOU CAN WRAP THE ROOT TIGHTLY IN PLASTIC AND FREEZE IT. REMOVE FROM FREEZER (DO NOT THAW), GRATE WHAT YOU NEED, AND RETURN THE REST TO THE COLD. FROZEN GINGER WILL KEEP ITS FLAVOR FOR ABOUT A MONTH.

spinach salad
with pine nut dressing

6 cups of spinach leaves, washed and carefully dried

1/4 cup pine nuts, chopped fine

1/4 cup olive oil

3 tablespoons tarragon vinegar

1/4 teaspoon grated lemon peel (optional)

1/2 teaspoon salt

Put spinach in a bowl. Combine remaining ingredients and pour over spinach. Toss gently.

Serves 6.

VEGAN, GLUTEN-FREE

SALADS MAKE THE MOST OF WINTER SPINACH, WHICH GENERALLY DOESN'T GROW FAST ENOUGH TO PROVIDE LARGE QUANTITIES FOR COOKING. THE TASTE IS A REVELATION, INCOMPARABLY SWEETER AND RICHER THAN THAT OF SUMMER VARIETIES. SUNFLOWER SEEDS WON'T GIVE THE SAME EFFECT AS PINE NUTS, BUT THEY ALSO MAKE A GOOD SALAD, AT A MUCH REDUCED PRICE.

turnip salad

1 pound small turnips

2 tablespoons sesame oil

1 teaspoon sugar

1/4 teaspoon ground ginger

2 tablespoons soy sauce

2 tablespoons cider vinegar

Peel turnips if necessary and cut into fine slivers. Mix with remaining ingredients and marinate for several hours.

Serves 6.

VEGAN

THE JAPANESE ARE GREAT CONNOISSEURS OF TURNIPS, GROWING MANY VARIETIES UNFAMILIAR IN NORTH AMERICA. SMALL CRISP ROOTS ARE WHAT YOU WANT FOR SALADS SUCH AS THESE. THE BASEBALL-SIZED SPECIMENS AT THE SUPERMARKET ARE TOO HOT AND TOO CORKY TO USE RAW. THIS SALAD IS ALSO GOOD MADE WITH KOHLRABI. USE A GOOD-QUALITY SOY SAUCE.

semi-thai salad

SALAD

**1 bunch watercress leaves
(about 1/2 cup, packed), stemmed**

1/2 cup fresh mint leaves

1/4 cup fresh cilantro leaves

4 to 6 leaves Bibb or other soft leaf lettuce

**1/2 pound julienned stir-fried beef or
1/2 pound julienned cold roast beef
or 8 grilled prawns**

1 small bunch radishes, halved and sliced

1 small red onion, sliced thin

DRESSING

**3 tablespoons mild vegetable oil
(not olive oil for this dish)**

2 tablespoons fresh lemon or lime juice

**1 tablespoon Thai fish sauce or
2 teaspoons Vietnamese fish sauce**

1/2 teaspoon sugar

1/2 teaspoon black pepper

1/4 teaspoon dried hot pepper flakes

⊰⊱ cook's note

Thai fish sauce (nam pla) is milder than the Vietnamese version (nuoc mam), so amounts should be adjusted according to the provenance.

Mix greens together and put them on a serving dish. Arrange beef, radishes and onions on top.

Put all dressing ingredients in a jar. Cover and shake until combined. Pour over salad just before serving and toss lightly. Dressing will keep a few days in the refrigerator.

Serves 4.

WHEN I WROTE THE FIRST EDITION, THIS SALAD WAS INTENDED AS A NON-THREATENING
INTRODUCTION TO BASIC THAI FLAVORS. IN THE TWENTY YEARS SINCE, THAI FOOD HAS
BECOME MAINSTREAM ENOUGH THAT THE STUDENTS AT THE RURAL HIGH SCHOOL WHERE
I TEACH REGULARLY DEBATE THEIR FAVORITE GREEN CURRY VENUES, AND FISH SAUCE IS ON
MOST EVERY GROCERY SHELF. SO THIS SALAD IS NO LONGER LIKELY TO BE REVELATORY,
BUT IT'S STILL VERY GOOD. IN SUMMER I WOULD DOUBLE THIS RECIPE AND MAKE IT
THE MAIN COURSE. IN COLD WEATHER IT GOES WONDERFULLY WITH A SOUP OR CURRY.

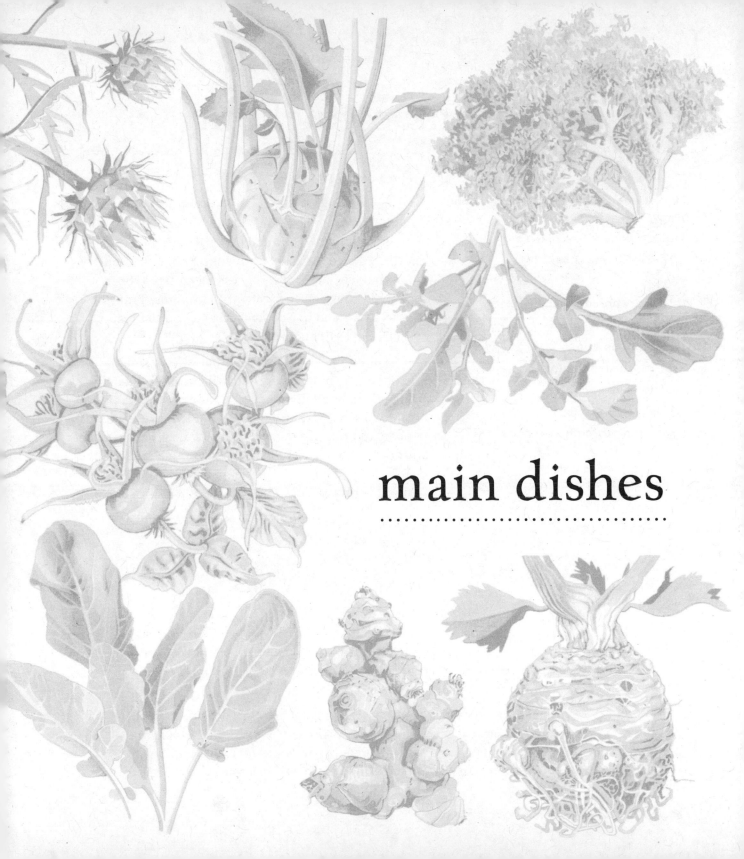

main dishes

hot pink cannelloni

12 cannelloni

1 baked beet, about 10 ounces (*see note below*)

5 tablespoons butter, divided

1/2 pound ricotta cheese

1 egg

1/2 cup dry bread crumbs

salt and pepper

2 tablespoons flour

1 cup milk or half-and-half

salt and white pepper

freshly grated nutmeg

1/3 cup grated Parmesan cheese

Preheat oven to 350°F.

Cook cannelloni in boiling salted water until almost tender. Drain and place on a lightly oiled plate, separating tubes so they don't stick together. Peel and slice the cooked beet. Purée until smooth. Melt 3 tablespoons of the butter in a saucepan. Add beet purée and cook gently for about 10 minutes. Transfer to bowl and blend in ricotta cheese, egg, and bread crumbs. Add salt and pepper to taste.

Melt remaining 2 tablespoons of butter in a small saucepan. Stir in flour and add milk or half-and-half. Bring just to boiling, reduce heat, and simmer gently until mixture is reduced to a sauce. Stir in salt, white pepper, and nutmeg to taste. While sauce is cooking, stuff cannelloni with beet mixture and place in lightly oiled baking dish, one layer deep. Pour sauce over and sprinkle with Parmesan cheese. Bake 30 minutes.

Serves 4.

VEGETARIAN

In Italy, vendors sell baked beets, ready to slice for salad with sweet onion, oil, and lemon or to use as a ravioli filling. I never seem to find the time to make ravioli, so I use the same beet mixture for cannelloni. The baked beets can also be served as is.

The cooked beets can be frozen for future use. Preheat oven to 350°F. Wrap each scrubbed but unpeeled beet in foil and bake until tender. Time will vary with the size of the beet, but count on at least 1½ hours, probably more. Do not undercook or the purée will be lumpy.

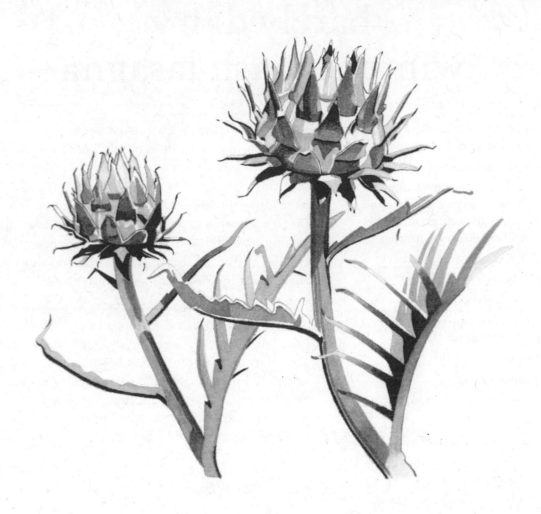

cardoons pellegrini

. . . .

barely dairy
winter squash lasagna

5 tablespoons olive oil, divided, or
4 tablespoons oil and one of butter

2 cloves garlic, chopped

2 cups sliced mushrooms (crimini,
portabella or a mixture of your choice;
I haven't tried this with chanterelles
but I'll bet it would be wonderful)

1/4 teaspoon salt

2 cups baked winter squash

up to 1/2 cup red wine

2 tablespoons chopped parsley or
mixed fresh Italian herbs

2 cups tomato sauce

3 tablespoons flour

2 cups unsweetened soy milk

salt and pepper

1/2 cup grated Romano cheese

1/4 pound mozzarella, grated or
sliced in thin strips

lasagna noodles (*see note below*)

Halve your squash with a cleaver, scoop out the strings and seeds, and rub a little olive oil onto the cut parts. Bake, skin side up, on a cookie tray in a 375°F oven until you can depress the flesh right through the skin. It's ok if some of the flesh blackens just a bit on the edges. (I use a silicon mat or bakers parchment to simplify cleanup.) Maybe 40 minutes, but it depends on the size and density of the squash. You can scoop the soft flesh right out of the skin with a serving spoon.

Heat 2 tablespoons of oil in a heavy saucepan or skillet, add the chopped garlic and cook for a minute or two. Don't let it brown. Add the sliced mushrooms and sauté until they start to get limp. Add squash and herbs, stir to mix in the mushrooms and garlic, and continue cooking over low heat for about 5 minutes. Add wine as needed to keep the mixture from sticking and stir occasionally. Remove from heat and reserve.

THIS SERVES 6 WITH LESS THAN ½ A POUND OF CHEESE TOTAL. YOU CAN SKIP THE CHEESE ENTIRELY, AND IT'S STILL GOOD, THOUGH THE FLAVOR BALANCE IS DIFFERENT. THE SECRET TO HAVING IT STILL DELIVER THE RICH, COMFORTING FEEL OF LASAGNA IS THE BÉCHAMEL. FOR REASONS I DON'T FULLY UNDERSTAND, UNSWEETENED SOY MILK MAKES A SUPERIOR BÉCHAMEL SAUCE. IT'S RICH AND CREAMY AND EVERY BIT AS SATISFYING AS A CREAM-BASED SAUCE. I DON'T FEEL THE SAME ABOUT SOY CHEESE, SOY MILK IN MY TEA, OR SOY YOGURT, BUT SOY BÉCHAMEL IS WORTH TRYING. THE SQUASH SHOULD BE A FLAVORFUL, DRY-FLESHED TYPE. I USED BUTTERNUT, BUT HUBBARDS, KABOCHAS, OR MANY OTHERS WOULD FILL THE BILL. I LEAVE IT TO YOU WHETHER TO PREBOIL THE LASAGNA NOODLES OR USE A NO-BOIL VARIETY, WITH ONE CAVEAT: THIS COMBINATION IS LESS LIQUID THAN MANY LASAGNAS, WHICH MEANS THAT NO-BOIL NOODLES CAN END UP A BIT CHEWY.

In a small, heavy saucepan, heat the remaining olive oil or oil and butter over medium heat. Add the flour and stir right away so it makes a smooth paste instead of clumps. Slowly add the soy milk, stirring constantly. Bring to mixture to just below boiling, lower heat, and cooking, stirring often, until it begins to thicken. Add Romano cheese, salt and pepper and keep over very low heat for another minute or so until cheese is melted.

Remove from heat.

Assembly

Start with a thin layer of tomato sauce, followed by a layer of pasta, and half the squash/mushroom mixture. Another layer of pasta, a little more tomato sauce, the remaining squash, topped with slices of mozzarella, and half the béchamel. The final layer of pasta is topped with the rest of the tomato sauce and the béchamel, swirled together.

Bake at 350 F, covered, until pasta is tender and flavors are blended.

Serves 6.

VEGETARIAN

polenta-stuffed cabbage

10-12 green cabbage leaves

4 to 5 tablespoons olive oil

2 medium onions, coarsely chopped

2-1/2 cups water

1-1/2 teaspoons salt

1 cup polenta

1/2 pound farmer's cheese

1/4 teaspoon black pepper

1 large onion, sliced thin

4 cloves garlic, minced

2 cups sauerkraut, drained (use the juice to make ciorba, page 71)

1 cup tomato juice

sour cream or yogurt, optional

Carefully separate the cabbage leaves and cut out the hard core. Cook them in a large pot of boiling, salted water until tender, about 5 minutes. Drain and reserve.

Sauté the onions in 2 tablespoons olive oil in a skillet or heavy saucepan until the onions caramelize to a golden brown. This can take up to 40 minutes. Stir and scrape often so the onions don't stick to the bottom and burn. When the onions are soft and sweet, add the water and salt to the pan and bring to a boil. Add the polenta slowly, stirring constantly. Turn down the heat and cook until the polenta is thick soft mush, about 15 minutes. Remove from heat, add cheese and pepper, and let cool.

Sauté the sliced onion and garlic in the remaining 2 tablespoons of oil in a large heavy skillet or Dutch oven, until the onion wilts and softens. It should not color up. Add the sauerkraut and tomato juice and mix well. Remove from heat while you make the cabbage rolls.

Place a spoonful of the cornmeal mixture (maybe a quarter cup, depending on the size of the leaves) on the middle of the cabbage leaf. Fold up the edges of the leaf over the filling and secure with a toothpick. Place the rolls on top of the sauerkraut mixture, one layer thick. Drizzle with a little olive oil. Bring to a simmer, cover, and cook for about an hour. More won't hurt.

Serve hot; pass around yogurt or sour cream as topping.

Serves 6.

GLUTEN-FREE

SUSPEND DISBELIEF. THIS UNUSUAL TREATMENT IS REALLY GOOD. IT COMES FROM ROMANIA, WHERE CABBAGE AND POLENTA (CALLED MAMALIGA) ARE BOTH STAPLES. LIKE ALL STUFFED CABBAGES, THERE IS A BIT OF LABOR INVOLVED, AND IT REHEATS WELL, SO DOUBLING THE RECIPE IS A GOOD IDEA. THE RECIPE IS ADAPTED FROM ELISABETH ROZIN'S FASCINATING BOOK, *CROSSROADS COOKING*. ANY MILD CHEESE WILL WORK HERE, BUT A CRUMBLY FARMER'S CHEESE IS JUST THE BEST.

root pot pie

6 cups vegetable stock or

6 cups water with 2 tablespoons vegetable bouillon base

10 cups root vegetables, peeled and cut in 1/2-inch cubes: carrots, celeriac, Hamburg parsley (sparingly), parsnips, turnips, small rutabagas

2 cups sweet winter squash or sweet potatoes, peeled and cubed into 1/2 inch cubes.

1 ounce dried mushrooms, broken into pieces, rinsed to remove grit, and soaked in 1 cup hot water for 1/2 hour I favor boletes (porcini), but any full-flavored fungus will work. To use 2 cups chopped fresh crimini or portabella mushrooms instead, skip the soaking.

3 tablespoons butter or oil

1 cup finely chopped onion or leek (white part only)

2–6 cloves garlic, chopped fine

salt and freshly ground pepper

1/2 cup flour

1/4 cup milk or soy milk

2 tablespoons dry sherry

1/4 cup chopped flat leaf parsley

Make dough for herbed biscuits (*see page 240*). Add 1/4 teaspoon minced fresh rosemary to biscuit recipe. Omit watercress.

Preheat oven to 400°F.

Bring stock to boil in large pot. Add root vegetables (not squash and/or yams) and simmer until vegetables are crisp/tender. Drain, reserve vegetables and broth in separate bowls.

Melt butter or heat oil in the same pot over medium heat. Add onions and sauté until they soften and begin to brown, perhaps 10 minutes depending on the water content of the onions. Mix in garlic and rosemary, stirring well. Add flour and stir thoroughly. Gradually whisk in reserved broth and then milk or soy milk and sherry. Cook gently until stock thickens and reduces to about 4 cups. Mix in reserved vegetables and parsley. Add salt and pepper. Spoon filling into a large heavy baking pan.

Bake, covered, for 50 minutes. Remove from oven, spoon biscuit batter over filling, and return to the oven and bake about 45 minutes, until biscuits are done. Cool slightly before serving.

Serves 10

VEGETARIAN

POT PIES ARE IDEAL FOR WINTER ROOTS, AND FOR THE NOT-QUITE-A-FULL-SERVING-OF-ANYTHING ISSUE COMMON TO SMALL WINTER GARDENS. THEY CAN BE TOPPED WITH PIE PASTRY, BISCUIT MIX, OR A SOFT POLENTA. I ADAPTED THIS VERSION FROM A RECIPE IN *BON APPETIT*. SKIPPING THE MEAT ALLOWS YOU TO EXPERIENCE THE VEGETABLE FLAVORS WITHOUT DISTRACTIONS.

spiced lentils and collard greens

2 tablespoons canola oil, butter, or niter kibbeh (*see page 231*)

1 medium onion, chopped fine

1 tablespoon finely chopped ginger root

4 cloves garlic, minced

2–3 fresh or frozen hot green chilies

1 cup lentils, rinsed and drained

2 cups water

1/2 pound trimmed collard greens, shredded or chopped (about 3 cups)

1 teaspoon ground cardamom

1 teaspoon salt

black pepper

yogurt

Heat oil or butter in a large heavy saucepan or skillet. Sauté onion, ginger, garlic, and chilies over medium heat until the vegetables soften, maybe 5 minutes. Add lentils, water, and collards. Bring to a simmer, and then cook over low to moderate heat, stirring occasionally, for about 20 minutes. Lentils should be tender but not dissolved into mush, and the whole mixture should be more like porridge than soup. Stir in cardamom, salt and pepper. Add hot sauce or sprinkle with cayenne if you like it hotter.

Pass yogurt on the side.

Serves 6.

VEGETARIAN, GLUTEN-FREE

THIS IS AN EAST AFRICAN COMBINATION FAMILIAR TO FANS OF ETHIOPIAN RESTAURANTS. THE BLEND OF STRONGLY FLAVORED GREENS, MELLOW LENTILS AND HOT SPICES MAKES A FEAST OUT OF PLAIN MATERIALS, AND A DAB OF YOGURT OR COTTAGE CHEESE ADDS A COOL COUNTERPOINT, RATHER LIKE THE INDIAN CURRY/RAITA PAIRING. DESPITE THEIR ASSOCIATION WITH TROPICAL CUISINES, HOT PEPPERS ARE MORE RELIABLE PRODUCERS IN COOL SUMMERS THAN ARE MOST SWEET VARIETIES. THEIR SMALLER SIZE AND THINNER FLESH REQUIRE LESS SUN AND HEAT TO DEVELOP. MY FRIEND MARY JEAN PRESERVES HER HOT PEPPERS FROM THE GARDEN BY REMOVING THE SEEDS AND FREEZING THEM ON TRAYS. THEY STAY IN FREEZER BAGS UNTIL NEEDED FOR COOKED RECIPES, AND THEY RETAIN THEIR FRESH TASTE ALTHOUGH NOT THEIR CRISP TEXTURE.

turkish cauliflower and lentil stew

1 medium to large cauliflower

4 tablespoons olive oil

1 cup finely chopped onion

1 carrot, chopped fine

2 garlic cloves, chopped fine

3 tablespoons chopped parsley

1 cup jerusalem artichoke (optional)

1 cup green or brown lentils

salt and pepper

1/4 teaspoon cayenne

1/2 cup chopped or ground canned Italian plum tomatoes, undrained

4 cups vegetable broth or water

Steam cauliflower until barely tender, 5 to 7 minutes. Drain and set aside. Heat oil in a saucepan. Add onion, carrot, garlic, parsley, and Jerusalem artichoke (if used), and sauté over medium heat for 5 minutes. Add lentils, salt, pepper, cayenne, and vegetable broth or water and wine and simmer, covered, stirring occasionally, until lentils are just tender, about 30 minutes.

Place tomatoes in a large saucepan; add cauliflower, lentils, and cooking liquid and simmer, covered, over very low heat for 30 minutes. Add water or broth during cooking as necessary, but do not stir the vegetables. Serve hot, sprinkled with a bit more parsley for garnish.

Serves 4 to 6.

VEGAN

TURKISH COOKING IS A LESSER-KNOWN TREASURE OF MEDITERRANEAN CUISINE. I'VE BEEN A FAN EVER SINCE A MEMORABLE FEW DAYS SPENT IN ISTANBUL IN THE 1960S, EATING BOUNTIFULLY FROM THE STREET CARTS FOR LESS THAN A DOLLAR A DAY. SINCE THEN I'VE EXPERIMENTED WITH A VARIETY OF RECIPES IN THE WONDERFUL BOOK, *CLASSICAL TURKISH COOKING*, BY AYLA ALGAR. THE ORIGINAL DISH, KARNIBAHAR MUSAKKA, USES GROUND MEAT INSTEAD OF LENTILS AND SKIPS THE ROOT VEGETABLES. THIS VARIATION IS ADAPTED FROM A VEGETARIAN VERSION CREATED BY PAOLA SCARAVELLI AND JON COHEN AND PUBLISHED IN *MEDITERRANEAN HARVEST*. MAYBE THAT'S TOO FAR FROM THE ORIGINAL TO STILL BE TRULY TURKISH, BUT IT'S VERY GOOD.

kale manicotti

2 large bunches kale, ribs removed

1 pound ricotta cheese

1 cup grated Parmesan cheese, divided

1 egg, lightly beaten

1 teaspoon minced garlic

2 teaspoons chopped parsley

1/2 teaspoon paprika

1 teaspoon fresh basil or 1/2 teaspoon dried

nutmeg, salt and white pepper to taste

1/2 pound fresh sheet pasta

1 cup tomato sauce

Preheat oven to 350°F.

Steam kale briefly, no more than 2 minutes. Remove from steamer, squeeze out excess moisture, and chop coarsely. Mix together in a large bowl ricotta cheese, 1/2 cup of the Parmesan cheese, egg, garlic, parsley, paprika, basil, nutmeg, salt, and white pepper. Add kale and mix well.

Cut sheet pasta into 4-inch squares. In a large pot of boiling water, cook pasta al dente, 3 or 4 minutes. Drain and rinse in cold water until cool enough to handle. Lay a pasta square on a kitchen towel. Pat dry. Using about 2 tablespoons of cheese mixture, lay filling diagonally across square. Bring opposite corners of square up across filling, pressing edges together to seal.

Put a thin layer of tomato sauce in a 9-by-13-inch baking pan. Carefully lay the manicotti in the pan and drizzle with more tomato sauce. Bake, covered, for about 25 minutes. Sprinkle with the remaining 1/2 cup of Parmesan cheese and serve.

Serves 4.

VEGETARIAN

KALE COMBINES NICELY WITH A MILD CHEESE LIKE RICOTTA. (IT ALSO IS GOOD SIMPLY STEAMED AND SERVED WITH BÉCHAMEL OR A DASH OF GOOD VINEGAR.) THIS SIMPLE MANICOTTI FILLING, WHICH I GOT FROM MY FRIENDS FRED AND LYNN BERMAN AT PAZTAZZA IN BELLINGHAM, ALSO COULD BE MADE WITH RAAB.

hazelnut, chard, and goat cheese filo pie

1/4 package filo pastry

3 medium leeks, white part only, sliced thin

3 tablespoons unsalted butter

2 cloves garlic, chopped fine

1 teaspoon finely chopped English thyme or 1/2 teaspoon dried

2 teaspoons finely chopped marjoram or 3/4 teaspoon dried

1/4 cup dry white wine

3 large bunches Swiss chard or spinach, leaves only, washed and shredded

1/2 pound creamy goat-milk cheese

2 eggs, beaten

3/4 cup melted clarified butter

1 cup roasted crushed hazelnuts

1 tablespoon chopped chives

1 tablespoon chopped fennel leaves

1 tablespoon chopped rosemary

Preheat oven to 350°F.

If using frozen filo, remove pastry from freezer and let thaw while making filling. When thawed, unfold dough and cut in half crosswise. Melt the 3 tablespoons of butter and sauté leeks for 2 or 3 minutes. Add garlic, thyme, marjoram, and white wine. Cook, covered, until leeks are soft. Add chard or spinach and cook, uncovered, until greens are wilted and liquid has reduced by half. Pour mixture into a bowl. Add goat cheese and eggs and mix thoroughly.

Mix together chopped chives, fennel, and rosemary. Brush a 9-by-13-inch pan with some of the melted clarified butter and place a sheet of filo on the bottom. Brush with butter and sprinkle with hazelnuts and mixed herbs. Continue layering with butter, herbs, and hazelnuts for 10 sheets. Spoon spinach and cheese mixture evenly across pan. Continue with layers of filo, butter, and herbs 10 more times. Brush final layer with butter. Sprinkle herbs on top. Bake 40 to 45 minutes, until well browned.

Serves 6.

VEGETARIAN

THE KITCHEN STAFF AT SOOKE HARBOUR HOUSE ON VANCOUVER ISLAND HAS MODIFIED A RECIPE BY STEWART BARNES TO MAKE THIS SAVORY VARIATION ON SPANAKOPITA. THEY USE RED-STEMMED RUBY CHARD. REGULAR GREEN CHARD OR THE TRADITIONAL SPINACH MAY BE SUBSTITUTED.

russian vegetable pie

PASTRY

1-1/4 cups flour

1 teaspoon salt

2 tablespoons butter

4 ounces cream cheese

FILLING

4 tablespoons oil, divided

3 cups shredded green or red cabbage
(1 small cabbage)

1 medium onion, chopped

2 cups sliced mushrooms

salt and pepper

1/2 teaspoon dried dill weed

1/4 teaspoon fresh thyme or
1/8 teaspoon dried

4 ounces softened cream cheese

Preheat oven to 400°F.

Pastry

Sift together flour and salt. Cut in butter until mixture is the size of peas. Work in cream cheese and form pastry into two balls, one twice as big as the other. Chill until vegetables are ready. Then roll out the bigger ball and line a 9- or 10-inch pie pan. Roll out the remaining ball for the top crust.

Filling

Heat 2 tablespoons of the oil in a large skillet or saucepan. Add cabbage and onion and sauté for 10 minutes. Heat remaining 2 tablespoons oil in another skillet or pan. Add mushrooms, salt, pepper, dill, and thyme and sauté for 5 minutes

Spread cream cheese in bottom of pie shell. Spread cabbage and onion mixture evenly over cream cheese and follow with mushrooms. Cover with top crust. Make some decorative cuts in the top crust. Bake 15 minutes at 400°F, reduce heat to 350°F, and bake another 20 to 25 minutes. Cool a few minutes before serving.

Serves 6.

VEGETARIAN

GREAT FOR LUNCH, THIS DISH MAKES PLAIN INGREDIENTS TASTE SPECIAL. VARIATIONS ARE JUST ABOUT INFINITE. YOU NEED SOME CREAM CHEESE, SOME MUSHROOMS, AND SOMETHING IN THE CABBAGE FAMILY, BUT OTHER ADDITIONS (COOKED CARROTS, CELERIAC, ALMONDS OR HAZELNUTS, STEAMED SALSIFY) AND SUBSTITUTIONS ARE WELCOME.

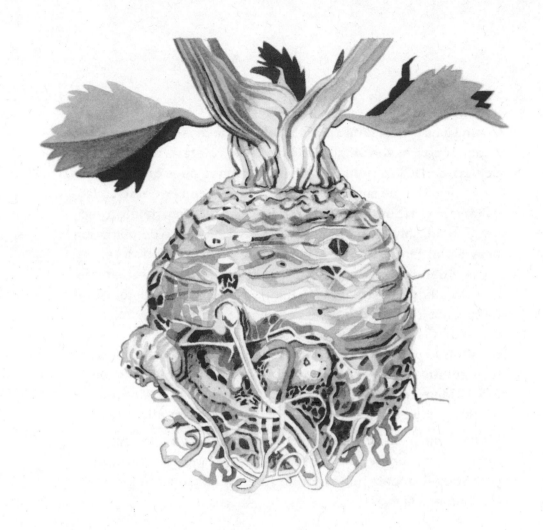

celeriac

....

PIZZAS

When I was a kid, I hated pizza. That was because my only experience was the version served in the cafeteria at Edgemont School, and it was right up there with canned peas on my personal no-go list. That all changed a decade later when I went to college in Italy for two quarters. I learned to love espresso, gelato, fried baby squid, shivering through the Uffizi Gallery in a combination of awe and January cold, rattling through the cobbled streets in my boyfriend's Fiat cinquecento…and pizza: Margharetta pizza, quattro staggioni pizza, crispy thin-crusted pizzas with real food on top, not lost in a swamp of bad cheese. Now I can get all of those things close to home, plus vegan pizza that's actually good, gluten-free pizza crusts, and no doubt other permutations I've yet to encounter. I've also learned that pizza is a winter gardener's friend. Many traditional regional specialties employ winter produce, and other combinations await your inspiration.

It's also much easier to find a variety of good premade crusts, but making your own pizza dough is simple, and you can indulge your show-biz fantasies by tossing and twirling it inches from the kitchen ceiling.

basic pizza dough

1 cup warm water

2 teaspoons dry yeast

1 teaspoon salt

4 tablespoons olive oil

2-3/4 cups bread flour

Put warm water in large bowl. Sprinkle yeast over the surface, let it sit for 3 or 4 minutes, and then mix. Add salt and oil and mix again. Stir in flour and begin kneading in the bowl. When the sticky dough begins to pull away from the sides of the bowl, turn onto a floured surface and knead until silky, another 10 or 12 minutes. Add as little flour as possible to get a manageable dough.

Return dough to a clean, lightly floured bowl. Cover with a kitchen towel and let rise in a warm, draft-free place until doubled in size, at least 2 hours. Punch down dough. (At this point you can refrigerate the dough for up to a day or freeze it in an airtight container for up to a month. Remove from refrigerator half an hour before using and from freezer 2 hours before using.) Separate dough into balls if you are making more than one pizza. Roll into desired shape. Dough should be no more than 1/4-inch thick. Place dough on ungreased pan, top, and bake.

*Makes 1 large or
8 individual pizzas.*

A FLAVORFUL OLIVE OIL GIVES THIS CRUST EXTRA PRESENCE.
THIS IS MY FAVORITE HOMEMADE CRUST.

campania pizza

20 cured Italian olives, pitted and coarsely chopped

4 tablespoons pine nuts

4 tablespoons raisins, coarsely chopped

2 tablespoons capers, coarsely chopped

1 medium head chicory or escarole

olive oil

8 anchovy fillets, chopped into small pieces

Preheat oven to 500°F.

Put chopped olives in a medium bowl. Brown pine nuts carefully in a bare skillet over medium-low heat. Don't let them burn. Add to olives, along with raisins and capers, and stir. Chop chicory or escarole roughly and boil in a small amount of water until tender, about 5 minutes. Drain chicory well (the cooking water is good in soup) and spread to cool. Once chicory is cool, wrap in a towel and squeeze out as much water as you can.

Cook anchovies briefly in about 2 tablespoons olive oil over medium heat. Add chicory and mix well. Use a bit more oil if necessary. Cook gently about 5 minutes. Let cool.

Roll out pizza dough to fit your pan. Drizzle on a little olive oil and then spread the anchovy and chicory mixture. Sprinkle on some salt and pepper and drizzle some more olive oil. Bake at bottom of oven for about 7 minutes. Serve hot.

Serves 6 to 8.

THIS HIGHLY FLAVORED TREAT IS TRADITIONAL TO THE CHRISTMAS SEASON IN THE SOUTHERN ITALIAN REGION OF CAMPANIA, WHICH IS ALSO HOME TO NAPLES, POMPEII, THE OLDEST KNOWN PIZZA PARLOR, AND THE LUSCIOUS SAN MARZANO TOMATO.

leek and olive pizza

pizza dough

3 tablespoons olive oil

6 medium leeks, chopped, with an inch of green

2 tablespoons chopped dried tomatoes (optional)

20 Italian olives, pitted and chopped

3 tablespoons Parmesan cheese

Preheat oven to 500°F.

Heat olive oil in a medium skillet. Add leeks and sauté gently for about 15 minutes. The leeks are taking the place of tomato sauce, so let them get really soft. Add dried tomatoes, if used, in the last 5 minutes of cooking. Spread mixture onto thin pizza dough. Sprinkle with chopped olives and Parmesan cheese and bake about 7 minutes on the bottom shelf.

Serves 4 to 6.

VEGETARIAN

PUNGENT OLIVES AND SWEET COOKED LEEKS COMBINE FOR A SIMPLE TOPPING. THE DRIED TOMATOES ARE A NICE TOUCH. I DRY SOME OF MY OWN EACH SUMMER IN A SIMPLE FOOD DRIER. (SEE OTHER INGREDIENTS SECTION OF PRODUCE LIST.)

vegan winter pizza

1/2 pound fresh mushrooms, sliced (I use crimini)

2 tablespoons chopped onion greens (scallions, garlic chives, small leeks, shallot greens, whatever the garden has on offer)

2 tablespoons olive oil, divided

2 pounds fresh spinach, stemmed and chopped, or 1 package frozen chopped spinach, thawed but not drained

2 teaspoons good quality vinegar (balsamic, muscat, or other vinegar with a touch of sweetness)

2 tablespoons gremolata (*see page 233*)

Dough for 9-inch pizza.

Preheat oven to 425°F. Warm 1 tablespoon of the olive oil, add mushrooms and onion greens, and sauté slowly until mushrooms get slippery. Stir in the spinach and cook at medium-low until moisture starts to evaporate. Sprinkle on the vinegar. Mix remaining tablespoon olive oil into the gremolata and add to the vegetables. Add salt and freshly ground pepper to taste, stir, and press the mixture down into a sort of patty. Cook until there is no free liquid but the spinach is still moist. It should have about the consistency of hummus.

Spread on pizza crust and bake about 15 minutes until crust is golden.

Serve warm. You could drizzle on a bit more olive oil to taste.

Serves 4 to 6.

VEGAN

Maybe 15 years ago, I visited friends in Massachusetts who introduced me to the world of vegan takeout, an oxymoron in rural Whatcom County at the time but not in Cambridge.

The roasted eggplant, tomato, and fresh basil pizza we had my first night was a revelation to me. It was vegan, it was wonderful, *and* it was delivered. I was also delighted that the pizza had nothing pretend—no non-dairy "cheese," no texturized vegetable protein. All the complementary tastes and textures that satisfy a pizza lover were created out of honest fresh vegetables. Since then I have learned a lot more about good vegan cooking, and I have come to appreciate the ways that knowledgeable cooks create rounded, complex flavors out of a more restricted range of ingredients.

I already was familiar with a number of traditional Christmas pizzas common to southern Italy, with chard and anchovies or salty olives. I like them a lot, but I also wondered if there is a way to create the softness that is part of pizza pleasure, with vegan winter garden ingredients. I think this combination does the trick. The spinach mixed with gremolata has the texture of a good tomato sauce. The mushrooms contrast with the greens, and the vinegar has the sweet tang that in summer would be a tomato's job.

linguine with broccoli, cauliflower, and mushrooms

1 cup ricotta cheese

1/3 cup grated Romano cheese

1 teaspoon salt

1 medium head broccoli, peeled and trimmed

1 medium head cauliflower, separated into florets

1/2 cup olive oil

6 cloves garlic, minced

1 pound mushrooms, sliced thin

2 teaspoons salt

1/2 teaspoon red pepper flakes

1 pound linguine

Combine ricotta and Romano cheeses in a small bowl and set aside. Add broccoli and cauliflower to boiling salted water in a large pot. Cook uncovered until vegetables are almost tender, about 5 to 7 minutes. Remove vegetables with slotted spoon. Keep liquid for cooking linguine.

Heat olive oil and garlic in a large, heavy skillet. When garlic is lightly browned, stir in mushrooms, salt, and red pepper flakes and sauté about 5 minutes. Stir in broccoli and cauliflower and continue cooking until vegetables are tender but not mushy (about 10 minutes). Add some of the cooking water if mixture seems too dry.

Bring cooking water to a rapid boil, adding more water if needed. Add linguine and cook, uncovered, about 10 to 12 minutes. Drain. Reheat vegetables. Stir in linguine, divide among shallow bowls, and top with cheese mixture and some more grated Romano cheese.

Serves 4 as a main dish or 6 as a first course.

VEGETARIAN

SIMPLE AND QUICK, THIS DISH COUNTS ON REALLY FRESH VEGETABLES FOR ITS FLAVOR. IF YOU GROW OVERWINTERED BROCCOLI AND CAULIFLOWER, IT CAN BE ONE OF THE FIRST TREATS OF SPRING.

haricot mélange

6 cups water

1/2 pound dry white beans or small limas

2-1/2 pounds Swiss chard (3 or 4 bunches), stems removed

1/4 cup olive oil

1 small onion, coarsely chopped

6 to 8 canned tomatoes, drained and coarsely chopped

3 medium cloves garlic, chopped

1/4 teaspoon dried basil

1/2 teaspoon fresh thyme or 1/4 teaspoon dried

salt and pepper

Bring water to boil in a saucepan, add beans, and boil 2 minutes. Remove from heat and let stand 1 hour. Return to boil, reduce heat, and simmer until beans are tender, about 1-1/2 hours. Drain.

Wash chard, shake off extra water, and cook in a large saucepan over high heat until wilted, 3 to 4 minutes. Stir frequently so it doesn't scorch. Drain well, squeeze dry, and chop coarsely.

Heat olive oil in heavy skillet over medium heat. Add onion and sauté until softened. Stir in beans, chard, tomatoes, garlic, basil, and thyme. Add salt and pepper to taste. Reduce heat and simmer 15 minutes to blend flavors, stirring frequently. Adjust seasoning and serve.

Serves 6.

VEGAN, GLUTEN-FREE

SIMPLE FLAVORS SIMMER INTO A SATISFYING HARMONY. THE TYPE OF BEANS MATTERS.
I TRIED THIS WITH PINTOS ONCE, AND IT JUST WASN'T THE SAME.

baked jerusalem artichokes with mushrooms

up to 1/2 cup dried porcini mushrooms (optional)

2 cups water, or light stock if no dried mushrooms are used

2 pounds Jerusalem artichokes, scrubbed

3 strips bacon or 2 tablespoons oil

1 onion, chopped

sliced mushrooms to total 2 cups with porcini

1/4 teaspoon nutmeg

1/4 teaspoon ginger

salt and pepper

1/2 cup grated Swiss cheese

1 tablespoon butter

Preheat oven to 450°F.

Soak dried mushrooms (if used) in water for an hour; remove mushrooms and slice. Pour mushroom water or stock into a saucepan, heat to boiling, and add artichokes. Simmer until artichokes are tender but not mushy. Drain artichokes, peel, and chop coarsely.

Fry bacon or heat oil in a medium skillet. Remove bacon (if used) and pour off excess drippings. Add chopped onion and sauté until it begins to soften. Add soaked and fresh mushrooms and sauté another 2 or 3 minutes. Combine artichokes, mushrooms, onions, bacon (if used), nutmeg, ginger, salt, and pepper in a medium bowl.

Grease a casserole with bacon grease or a little butter. Spread on a layer of artichokes and onion and sprinkle with grated Swiss cheese. Make additional layers, ending with cheese. Dot with butter and bake for about 20 minutes.

Serves 4.

THIS HAS A SWEET, EARTHY TASTE, WHICH WILL VARY WITH THE TYPE OF MUSHROOMS. IF YOU GATHER YOUR OWN, YOU CAN USE NORTHWEST BOLETUS EDULUS, FRESH OR DRIED; THEY'RE THE SAME SPECIES AS THE PRICEY PORCINI.

broccoli dal curry

1 cup lentils

4 tablespoons ghee (*see page 236*) or
light oil

2 medium onions, chopped fine

1 teaspoon chili powder

2 teaspoons black pepper

1-1/2 teaspoons ground cumin

1-1/2 teaspoons ground coriander seeds

2 teaspoons turmeric

juice of half a lemon

2 medium heads broccoli

2 cups water

1/2 cup unsweetened dried coconut

1 tablespoon flour

1 teaspoon salt

1 cup cashews or peanuts

⊰⊱ cook's note

If you are using the small side shoots that overwintered plants sprout in the spring, reduce the steaming time to keep them crisp-tender.

Wash lentils well and drain. Heat ghee or oil in a large saucepan and sauté onions until they begin to soften. Add chili powder, black pepper, cumin, coriander, and turmeric. Stir and cook briefly. Add lentils, stir well, and add lemon juice, water, and coconut. Bring to a boil, reduce heat, and simmer about 25 to 30 minutes or until lentils are soft.

Meanwhile, cut broccoli into individual florets. (Save stems for another use.) Steam 5 or 10 minutes, until almost tender. Plunge broccoli in cold water, drain, and set aside.

Remove 1/3 cup of liquid from the lentil mixture, add to flour to form a smooth paste, and return it to the pan. Add steamed broccoli, salt, and nuts. Simmer another 5 to 10 minutes, until the lentils make a thick sauce. Serve with basmati rice.

Serves 4.

VEGETARIAN, GLUTEN-FREE

I LIKE THE SMALLER INDIAN LENTILS (DAL) IN THIS DISH—BROWN, YELLOW, OR PINK—
BUT IT'S FINE WITH THE REGULAR GROCERY STORE TYPES. GOOD FRESH BROCCOLI,
NOT OVERCOOKED, IS MUCH MORE IMPORTANT.

spicy squash stew
with cornmeal dumplings

1 cup sliced onion

4 tablespoons olive oil

6 cloves garlic, peeled and minced

3/4 teaspoon ground cumin

3/4 teaspoon cinnamon

3/4 cup diced, seeded hot green chilies
(adjust amount and firepower to your
taste)

7 cups (two 28-ounce cans) canned
tomatoes

1 pound winter squash, peeled and cut
into 1/2-inch cubes

1-1/2 teaspoons salt

1-1/2 cups water

1/2 pound mushrooms, quartered

3 tablespoons chopped cilantro

DUMPLINGS

1 cup yellow cornmeal

1/3 cup white flour

1 teaspoon baking powder

3/4 teaspoon salt

1 teaspoon sugar

1 egg

1/2 cup half-and-half or milk

1-1/2 tablespoons melted butter

Sauté onion in olive oil in a large, wide pot until transparent. Add garlic, cumin, cinnamon, and chilies. Sauté a few minutes more, stirring constantly. Chop tomatoes coarsely and add them with their liquid, squash, salt, and water. Lower heat, cover pot, and simmer gently for about 1 hour. Add mushrooms and cilantro and simmer another 5 minutes. Drop dumpling batter (see recipe below) on stew by teaspoonfuls, cover pot tightly, and simmer over very low heat for 20 minutes.

Dumplings

Sift together cornmeal, flour, baking powder, salt, and sugar. Beat together egg and half-and-half or milk and stir into dry mixture. Add melted butter and stir until batter is smooth. Add to stew right away, and serve as soon as dumplings are done.

Makes 2 dozen dumplings.

Serves 6 to 8.

VEGETARIAN

A VARIATION ON A RECIPE FROM ANNA THOMAS'S *VEGETARIAN EPICURE*, BOOK TWO,
THIS COMBINES FAMILIAR MEXICAN FLAVORS IN A FRESH AND DELICIOUS WAY.
ALL IT NEEDS IS A SALAD AND MAYBE A BEER.

nettle omelet

4 cups nettle leaves, loosely packed
(See note below.)

1/2 cup ricotta cheese

5 tablespoons butter, divided

2 shallots, minced, or 2 tablespoons
minced onion

5 eggs, beaten

salt and pepper

pinch of fresh tarragon (optional)

Steam nettle leaves until limp. Remove from heat, press out moisture, and chop. Mix with ricotta cheese and set aside. Melt 1 tablespoon butter in a small saucepan, add shallots or onion, cook gently until they start to turn color, and stir them into nettle mixture. Add salt and pepper to beaten eggs. Melt remaining butter in an omelet pan or your closest approximation. Add eggs and cook over low heat, loosening edges as they solidify and letting uncooked egg run under. Spoon ricotta cheese-nettle mixture onto one half of the omelet, leaving a 2-inch margin bare. Slide a spatula gently under the other half and fold omelet over filling. Cook very gently, about 2 minutes on each side, sprinkle with tarragon (if used), and serve hot.

Serves 2 or 3.

VEGETARIAN, GLUTEN-FREE

AROUND HERE, HOMESTEAD CHICKENS COME OUT OF THEIR WINTER EGG-LAYING SLUMP ABOUT THE TIME THE NEW NETTLE CROP IS 3 OR 4 INCHES TALL. THIS MAKES NETTLE OMELETS A SPRING RITUAL. WEAR RUBBER GLOVES WHEN HARVESTING AND PREPARING NETTLES AND USE THE LEAVES ONLY. (FOR MORE ON NETTLES, SEE PAGE 26.)

sunday brunch frittata

3 tablespoons cup light oil

2 leeks, with some green, trimmed and sliced into thin rounds

3 medium Jerusalem artichokes, scrubbed and sliced thin

1/2 cup parsley, chopped

2 tablespoons fresh cilantro

1 teaspoon dried basil

6 eggs

1/3 cup milk

1/3 cup sour cream

salt and pepper

1 cup grated Muenster or Monterey Jack cheese

Heat oil in a large skillet and sauté leeks and Jerusalem artichokes over medium-low heat until soft, 5 to 7 minutes. Add parsley, cilantro, and basil and sauté 2 more minutes. Remove mixture from the pan and set aside.

Beat eggs in medium bowl. Beat in milk, sour cream, salt, and pepper. Return skillet to burner and heat to medium. Add egg mixture and reduce heat to low. Spread vegetable mixture evenly over eggs and cover with cheese.

Cook gently until eggs have set on bottom and top is just slightly soupy. Place skillet under broiler with door ajar and cook until top is golden and puffy. Serve at once.

Serves 3 or 4.

VEGETARIAN, GLUTEN-FREE

THIS DISH IS THE PERFECT ANTIDOTE TO TOO MUCH WHOLESOME OATMEAL. THE SMALLER THE PAN, THE THICKER AND PUFFIER THE RESULT AND THE LONGER THE COOKING TIME. PURISTS MIGHT WANT TO TURN THE ALMOST-FINISHED FRITTATA ONTO A PLATE AND THEN SLIDE IT BACK UPSIDE-DOWN INTO THE PAN FOR THE LAST MINUTE OF COOKING. I FIND IT EASIER TO FINISH IT UNDER THE BROILER, WHICH ALSO MEANS THAT I CAN SHOW OFF THE DECORATIVE PATTERN OF VEGETABLES ON TOP.

indian spinach with potatoes

2 pounds boiled peeled potatoes

1 pound fresh spinach

1/4 cup peanut or other light oil

1 cup chopped onion

1 or 2 cloves garlic, minced

1-inch piece fresh ginger, peeled and sliced thin

1 teaspoon mustard seed

1 teaspoon ground cumin

red pepper flakes (optional)

1 teaspoon turmeric

1/2 teaspoon chili powder

1 teaspoon salt, or to taste

Cut potatoes into cubes. You should have about 4 cups. Chop spinach coarsely. Heat oil in a large saucepan, add onion, garlic, and fresh ginger, and sauté briefly. Combine mustard seed, cumin, red pepper flakes (if used), turmeric, and chili powder. Add to saucepan, stir well, and cook mixture over gentle heat until onion is soft.

Add potatoes and stir gently to coat them with spices. Add spinach in handfuls. Add salt, stir again carefully but thoroughly, cover, and cook 3 minutes or so, until spinach is cooked down a bit. Serve at once.

Serves 4 to 6.

VEGAN, GLUTEN-FREE

THIS IS QUICK AND GOOD. IF YOU BOIL THE POTATOES BEFOREHAND, YOU CAN HAVE DINNER ON THE TABLE IN ABOUT 10 MINUTES. YOU CAN ADJUST THE SPICINESS ACCORDING TO THE TYPE OF CHILI POWDER YOU USE, AND BY THE ADDITION OF RED PEPPER FLAKES. SERVE WITH CARROT CURRY (*SEE PAGE 170*) AND A RAITA (*SEE PAGE 95*) FOR A BEAUTIFUL AND NUTRITIOUS VEGETARIAN MEAL. THE ¼ CUP OF OIL SEEMS LIKE A LOT, BUT IT IS NEEDED TO COAT THE POTATOES.

chard tart

1 pound Swiss chard

lemon juice

2 tablespoons olive oil

1 medium onion, chopped fine

2 cloves garlic, chopped fine

salt and pepper

freshly grated nutmeg

1-1/2 cups ricotta cheese

1/2 cup plus 1 tablespoon Parmesan cheese, divided

1/2 cup milk

3 eggs, beaten

partially baked pastry shell

Preheat oven to 350°F.

Remove chard stems, wash leaves, and blanch 2 to 3 minutes in salted water with a squeeze of lemon. Leaves should be tender but still bright green. Drain, rinse with cold water, squeeze dry, and chop into shreds.

Heat olive oil in a medium skillet. Add onion and sauté a few minutes. Do not let it brown. Add chard and garlic and cook over medium-high heat for 5 minutes or until moisture is absorbed. Be careful that it doesn't scorch. Sprinkle with salt, pepper, and nutmeg and remove from heat.

Stir ricotta cheese in mixing bowl. Add milk, beaten eggs, and 1/2 cup of the Parmesan cheese and blend until smooth. Stir in chard mixture and adjust seasoning.

Pour into pastry shell, sprinkle with remaining Parmesan cheese, and bake about 40 minutes. Cool slightly before serving.

Serves 6.

VEGETARIAN

THIS MEATLESS VERSION OF JUDIE GEISE'S RECIPE IN *THE NORTHWEST KITCHEN* TASTES RICHER THAN IT IS, AND THE GREEN-FLECKED, GOLDEN PIE IS ATTRACTIVE. IT IS A GOOD USE FOR SOMEWHAT WEATHER-BEATEN WINTER CHARD.

feijoada

BEANS

1 large onion, chopped

2 cloves garlic, chopped

oil

1 cup dry black (turtle) beans

3 cups stock (or substitute white wine for half the stock)

1 bay leaf

salt and pepper

1 whole peeled orange

2 stalks celery or Swiss chard stems, chopped

1 canned tomato, drained and chopped

RICE

1 onion, chopped

3 cloves garlic, minced

2 tablespoons vegetable oil

2 tablespoons butter or lard

2 canned tomatoes, drained, seeded and chopped

2 cups cooked rice

Beans

Sauté onion and garlic in a little oil in a deep, heavy pot. Add beans, cover with stock, and add bay leaf. Bring to a boil, simmer 2 minutes, turn off heat, and let stand, covered, for an hour. Add orange, celery or chard, tomato, salt, and pepper. Bring back to a boil and simmer, covered, for 2 to 3 hours, until beans are tender. Remove a ladleful of beans, mash them, and return to the pot. Cook gently, stirring often, until mixture begins to thicken.

Rice

Sauté onion and garlic in oil and butter until golden. Add tomatoes and cooked rice and warm over low heat.

A REAL BRAZILIAN FEIJOADA IS A MAJOR PROJECT. IT REQUIRES DRIED BEEF, SMOKED TONGUE, HOT SAUSAGE, SALT PORK, AND A LONG SIESTA AFTERWARDS. THE VEGETARIAN VERSION PRESENTED BY FRANCES MOORE LAPPÉ IN *DIET FOR A SMALL PLANET* IS MUCH SIMPLER TO MAKE AND PROBABLY CLOSER TO WHAT IS EATEN OUTSIDE THE MOST AFFLUENT CIRCLES. I LOVE IT. YOU CAN USE LARD OR BACON DRIPPINGS INSTEAD OF OIL AND COOK THE BEANS IN BEEF STOCK IF YOU WANT A MORE AUTHENTIC FLAVOR. THIS IS A COMPLETE MEAL. FINISH IT OFF WITH SOME STRONG, SWEET COFFEE AND A FLAN IF YOU WANT TO MAINTAIN A BRAZILIAN FEEL.

SALSA

1 frozen tomato (see Other Ingredients section of Produce List), thawed and skinned

1 jalapeno or other hot green pepper, seeded (more if you like it hot)

1 teaspoon salt

2 cloves garlic, crushed

juice of 1 lemon

1 small onion, chopped

1 tablespoon finely chopped cilantro or parsley

2 green onions or equivalent amount of chives, chopped

1/4 cup red wine vinegar

GREENS

1-1/2 pounds sturdy greens, trimmed and coarsely chopped (collards are traditional)

1 clove garlic, minced

1 tablespoon olive oil

4 tablespoons toasted sesame seeds

1 orange, peeled and sliced

Salsa

Put the tomato, hot green pepper, salt, and garlic in a blender and purée. Pour into serving bowl, add remaining ingredients, and stir. Just before serving, stir in a little liquid from the bean pot.

Greens

Steam greens until tender. (Time will vary according to what kind of greens you use.) Meanwhile, sauté garlic in olive oil. Add steamed greens and sauté, stirring, for no more than a minute. Put mixture in serving dish, sprinkle with sesame seeds, and arrange orange slices on top.

To Serve

Bring the four dishes separately to the table. Diners can start with a layer of rice, put a scoop of beans and their broth on top and some greens on the side, and top the lot with salsa to taste.

Serves 4.

VEGETARIAN

sorrel and leek bake

4 eggs

1/2 teaspoon salt

1/4 teaspoon pepper

1-1/2 cups water

1 cup yellow cornmeal

1 pound French sorrel or 3/4 pound wild sorrel, coarsely chopped

1 pound leeks (about 4 medium), white part only, sliced thin

3/4 cup grated Swiss cheese

5 tablespoons olive oil, divided

2 tablespoons grated Parmesan cheese

Preheat oven to 375°F.

Beat eggs in a small bowl until light. Add salt and pepper. In a medium bowl, add cold water gradually to cornmeal, stirring constantly until it is well mixed. Stir in eggs, and then stir in sorrel, leeks, and Swiss cheese.

Grease a large, shallow casserole or baking dish with 2 tablespoons of the oil. Pour in vegetable mixture, level top, and sprinkle with Parmesan cheese. Dribble remaining oil on top. Bake 50 to 60 minutes until set.

Serves 3 as a main dish or 4 as a side dish.

VEGETARIAN, GLUTEN-FREE

THE FIRST SPRING SORREL COMES UP WHILE OVERWINTERED LEEKS ARE STILL IN THEIR PRIME. THIS SWISS-ITALIAN DISH WAS NO DOUBT A GARDENER'S CREATION.

italian spinach and rice pie

3-1/2 cups chicken broth

two 10-ounce packages frozen spinach or 3 pounds fresh

4 tablespoons olive oil

1/2 cup pancetta or blanched bacon, chopped

1/4 cup chopped onion

1 large clove garlic, chopped

1 cup rice, preferably arborio or other short-grained variety

2 tablespoons butter

1/3 cup dry bread crumbs

4 eggs

1/2 cup grated Parmesan cheese

1 teaspoon dried marjoram

1/2 teaspoon freshly grated nutmeg

salt and pepper

Simmer broth over low heat. If you are using frozen spinach, it's easier to chop when partially thawed. Continue thawing, pressing excess moisture into heated broth. If you are using fresh spinach, steam leaves until soft, about 2 minutes. Remove from heat, chop, and press excess moisture into broth. Heat olive oil in large skillet over medium heat and sauté pancetta or bacon, onion, and garlic for 5 to 10 minutes. Mix in rice and cook 2 to 3 minutes, stirring constantly.

Reduce heat, stir in spinach, and bring to slow simmer. Cook, covered, adding broth 1/2 cup at a time, stirring frequently and allowing rice to absorb broth before adding more. This will take about 20 to 25 minutes. Rice should be creamy. Remove cover and let cool to room temperature.

Preheat oven to 350°F. Butter a 9-inch quiche dish or pie plate and sprinkle with bread crumbs. Shake off excess crumbs and reserve for topping.

Combine eggs, Parmesan cheese, marjoram, nutmeg, salt, and pepper in a large mixing bowl and beat well. Stir in rice mixture. Taste and adjust seasoning. Spoon into quiche dish or pie plate, spreading evenly. Sprinkle top with remaining bread crumbs. Bake until firm but not dry, about 45 minutes to 1 hour. Cool before serving.

Serves 5 as a main dish or 8 as a side dish.

A SIMPLE RISOTTO IS BAKED WITH EGGS IN A CRUMB CRUST. THE RESULT SLICES WELL AND IS EXCELLENT FOR POTLUCKS AND TAILGATE PICNICS. IF YOU HAVE LOTS OF TOP-QUALITY FRESH SPINACH, BY ALL MEANS USE IT.

kale, bacon, and potatoes

lean bacon strips

potatoes

kale

salt and pepper to taste

Amounts are approximate, but start with enough bacon for one layer in the skillet; and three times as much kale as potatoes by volume.

Line the bottom of a heavy skillet with bacon. Cover bacon with a layer of potatoes, which can be left whole if they are small, or quartered or sliced if they are larger. Wash kale, shake off excess water but do not dry and chop. Cram in as much chopped kale as will fit on top of the potatoes. Cover and cook very slowly over low heat. Check after an hour. The bacon and potatoes should be crisp, and the kale should be soft in the middle of the pan and a little crisp around the edges.

Servings depend on the size of your pan.

GLUTEN-FREE

THIS IS TRUE TRADITIONAL FARMERS' FOOD, POPULAR AMONG THE MANY DUTCH FAMILIES IN RURAL WHATCOM COUNTY. PREPARATION TIME IS ABOUT 1 MINUTE, THERE ARE NO EXTRA POTS AND PANS TO WASH, AND IT TASTES GREAT. IF YOU THINK IT SOUNDS TOO HEAVY, YOU'VE PROBABLY NEVER SPENT A DAY TENDING LIVESTOCK IN A JANUARY NORTHEASTER. IT'S AN EXCELLENT CHOICE FOR TOUGH OLD KALE. USED THICK-SLICED BACON; AROUND HERE THE BEST IS FROM HEMPLER'S. THIN-SKINNED POTATOES CAN BE LEFT UNPEELED.

romeo conca's
pork chops and kale

kale

1 pork chop per diner

black pepper

salt

olive oil

garlic, chopped, 1 clove for every 2 chops

꩜ cook's note

This recipe was created for the thicker, more marbled pork chops that were standard 20 years ago. If you are using the thinner, leaner ones common today, you need to make some adjustments. Sear the chops on one side only, and reduce cooking time. Check for doneness after 5 minutes. Very thin, very lean chops may cook too fast for the kale. In that case, blanch or steam the kale to soften it before adding to the pan.

Wash kale and remove any heavy stems. Pat pork chops dry. Dust one side lightly with dry mustard and grind on some pepper.

Coat the bottom of a heavy skillet with olive oil and heat to the smoking point. Salt the spiced side of the chops and cook, seasoned side down, until lightly browned. Salt top sides and turn.

Reduce heat to medium-low and cook until chops feel firm to the touch. Sprinkle in garlic and add as much as will fit in the pan. You can really cram it in. Drizzle in a little more olive oil and cover with a tight-fitting lid. Lower heat to simmer and cook until kale is limp. Cooking time will vary with the maturity of the kale.

GLUTEN-FREE

ROMEO WAS A CHEMIST WHO RETIRED TO FOUND AND RUN LOST MOUNTAIN WINERY ON WASHINGTON'S OLYMPIC PENINSULA. HE WAS ALSO A WONDERFUL COOK. HE ONCE DEBONED AN ENTIRE THANKSGIVING TURKEY AND FILLED THE CAVITIES WITH HOMEMADE SAUSAGE, SO THAT REASSEMBLED CREATURE COULD BE CARVED STRAIGHT ACROSS LIKE A LOAF OF BREAD. THAT MADE A MAJOR IMPRESSION ON ME AS A CHILD. BUT HE ALSO APPRECIATED SIMPLE SEASONAL DISHES, AND HE TOOK AN INTEREST IN THIS BOOK FROM THE START. HE SENT ME THIS RECIPE, WHICH IS DELICIOUS AND EASY AND JUST ABOUT FOOLPROOF AS LONG AS YOU ADJUST AS NECESSARY FOR LEANER CUTS OF MEAT.

italian sausage with fennel, carrot, and cabbage

1 cup dry white wine

1-1/2 to 2 pounds Italian link sausages

1 medium onion, minced

1 large carrot, julienned

4 cups coarsely chopped cabbage

2 large fennel bulbs, sliced thin

3 tablespoons minced fennel leaves, divided

1 garlic clove, minced

1/2 cup water

salt and pepper

Bring wine to boil in a large, heavy skillet. Prick each sausage in several places with fork and add to skillet. Reduce heat, cover, and simmer gently for 15 minutes. Remove cover and continue simmering until wine has evaporated. Then increase heat and brown sausage quickly. Remove sausages and keep warm.

Pour off all but 4 or 5 tablespoons fat from skillet. Turn heat to medium-high. Add onion and carrot and cook, stirring often, about 5 minutes. Stir in cabbage, sliced fennel, 2 tablespoons of the fennel leaves, garlic, and water. Cover and cook until vegetables are barely tender, about 3 to 5 minutes. Remove cover and boil off any liquid remaining in skillet. Remove from heat and adjust seasoning.

Make a bed of the vegetables on a serving platter. Arrange sausages on top, sprinkle with remaining fennel leaves, and serve.

Serves 4 to 6.

GLUTEN-FREE

red cabbage and chestnuts

20 fresh chestnuts

1/4 pound lean bacon or smoked sausage, diced

2 pounds red cabbage, shredded coarsely

3 cups beef stock

salt and pepper

Preheat oven to 375°F.

Cut an X in each chestnut shell and simmer for 10 to 15 minutes in a covered saucepan. Remove from heat, drain, and peel. Chop roughly. Stew bacon or sausage in a small skillet, pouring off excess fat. Place cabbage and bacon or sausage in a large ovenproof casserole, add stock and chestnuts, and season to taste with salt and pepper. Stir gently, cover, and cook until tender, about 1-1/2 hours.

Serves 4 to 6.

GLUTEN-FREE

THIS DISH IS FROM LIMOGES IN CENTRAL FRANCE. THE CHESTNUTS SOAK UP
THE RICH BLEND OF FLAVORS DURING A SLOW COOKING.

pot roast
with hazelnut barley

1 tablespoon olive oil

3- to 4-pound boneless chuck or other lean roast

2 medium onions, chopped fine

2 cloves garlic, chopped

2 tablespoons Dijon mustard

1 teaspoon fresh tarragon or 1/2 teaspoon dried

2 canned tomatoes, drained and chopped

salt and pepper

2 tablespoons butter

1/2 cup finely chopped hazelnuts

3 cups water

1 teaspoon salt

1 teaspoon Worcestershire sauce

1-1/2 cups pearl barley

Heat olive oil in a heavy pan. Brown roast over medium heat. Add onion and garlic and cook until they begin to soften. Add mustard, tarragon, tomatoes, salt, and pepper. Cover pan, lower heat, and simmer until roast is tender, 1-1/2 to 2 hours. You don't need any other liquid.

During the last 40 minutes of cooking, melt butter in a heavy saucepan. Add hazelnuts and cook over medium-high heat until they are crisp and brown. Add water, salt, Worcestershire sauce, and barley. Cover and steam over low heat until water is absorbed, about 30 minutes.

Remove meat, slice, and serve with barley and pan juices.

Serves 6.

A VERSION OF THIS HEARTY DINNER WAS THE WINNER IN A WASHINGTON STATE CONTEST FOR BEEF RECIPES MANY YEARS AGO. ONE FOOD WRITER AT THE TIME SNIFFED THAT IT JUST WASN'T VERY NOUVELLE, BUT THE PROOF IS IN THE EATING. TENDER MEAT, A TANGY SAUCE, AND A CHEWY BARLEY-NUT MIXTURE MAKE A MEMORABLE MEAL WITH A MINIMUM OF FUSS. IT IS AN IDEAL TREATMENT FOR OLDER, LEANER MEATS. I HAVE SINCE MADE IT WITH A CHUNK OF MOOSE BROUGHT DOWN FROM ALASKA BY A FRIEND, WHO SOMETIMES HUNTS TO SUPPLY POTLATCH FEASTS, AND I'M SURE IT WOULD BE SUPERB WITH BISON.

curry beef
with cauliflower

1 pound round steak or rib steak

1 medium cauliflower, broken into florets

juice of 1 lemon

1 teaspoon salt

1 teaspoon black pepper

3 tablespoons ghee (*see page 236*) or light cooking oil

1 large onion, sliced thin

2 cloves garlic, sliced thin

2-inch piece fresh ginger, sliced

1-1/2 teaspoon chili powder (omit if using curry powder)

1 teaspoon ground turmeric (omit if using curry powder)

1 teaspoon ground cumin

1/2 cup yogurt

beef stock

2 teaspoons garam masala (*see page 235*) or curry powder

1 tablespoon fresh cilantro

Trim fat from beef, pound to tenderize, and cut into strips 1/2-inch wide. Sprinkle with lemon juice, salt, and black pepper. Marinate, covered, for at least 2 hours. Drain beef, saving marinade. Heat ghee or oil and sauté beef until it colors. Remove from pan and set aside. Add onion and garlic and sauté until soft. Add fresh ginger, chili powder, turmeric, and cumin and cook another 2 minutes.

Spoon in yogurt and cook 3 or 4 minutes. Add cauliflower florets and stir to coat. Add enough beef stock to the marinade to make 1-1/2 cups. Return beef to pan and cook over low heat, covered, until cauliflower is barely tender, about 10 to 12 minutes. Stir in garam masala or curry powder, sprinkle cilantro on top, and simmer another 5 minutes.

Serves 4.

BEEF CURRIES ARE RARE BECAUSE HINDUS ARE VEGETARIANS AND MUSLIM CUISINES FOCUS ON LAMB AND CHICKEN. THIS ONE IS FROM THE PORTUGUESE CHRISTIAN COMMUNITY OF GOA, ON THE WEST COAST OF INDIA. IT MAKES GOOD USE OF LESS-THAN-TENDER STEAK. IF YOU ARE USING CURRY POWDER INSTEAD OF GARAM MASALA, OMIT THE CHILI POWDER AND TURMERIC.

stew with squash

1 pound peeled winter squash or pumpkin

3/4 pound beef or pork stew meat

1/2 cup red wine

3-1/2 cups water or broth

salt to taste

3 garlic cloves chopped

1 cup canned tomatoes, drained and chopped

1 tablespoon tomato paste

2 tablespoons lemon juice

1 tablespoon chopped fresh mint leaves or 2 teaspoons dried

Cut squash into 1-inch cubes and set aside. Combine meat, water, and salt in a large pot. Bring to a boil and cook for 2 minutes, removing any scum that rises. Add garlic, tomatoes, tomato paste, and lemon juice. Lower heat and simmer, covered, for 1 hour. Add pumpkin and cook, covered, until pumpkin is soft, about 45 minutes. Stir in mint leaves just before serving.

Serves 4.

THE MINT HELPS GIVE THIS SIMPLE STEW AN UNEXPECTED FRESHNESS. CHOSE A FULL-FLAVORED SQUASH LIKE WALTHAM OR KUBOTA, SINCE IT IS A MAJOR PART OF THE TASTE. COOKING TIME WILL VARY WITH THE MEAT AND THE TYPE AND AGE OF THE SQUASH. YOU WANT THE MEAT TO BE TENDER, OF COURSE, AND THE SQUASH CUBES TO BE SOFT BUT NOT DISSOLVED INTO PURÉE. SERVE OVER RICE OR WITH A PILAF ON THE SIDE.

gobo wrapped with beef

3/4 pound very lean boneless beef

1/4 cup soy sauce

1/4 cup mirin or sweet sherry

3/4 pound gobo (burdock)

4 cups water

1 tablespoon vinegar

Cut beef into thin slices across the grain. Mix soy and mirin or sherry in a small saucepan and heat until warm. Remove from heat; add beef and let stand at least 30 minutes. Scrub and peel gobo, cut into 5-inch lengths, and julienne. Bring water and vinegar to boil, add gobo, cover, reduce heat, and cook until just tender (about 5 minutes). Drain and cool enough to handle.

Holding 4 or 5 gobo strips in a bundle, wrap a beef strip spirally around bundle, covering the gobo. Use a second, overlapping strip if necessary. Stretch meat slightly as you go. Squeeze bundle to press meat firmly to gobo and then return to marinade.

When all bundles are made, remove from marinade and broil or grill. Cook, turning as needed, until lightly browned, 3 or 4 minutes. Cut each bundle into bite-sized pieces.

Serves 3 or 4 as a main course or 8 as an appetizer.

THIS TRADITIONAL JAPANESE DISH USES THE SAME CROSS-GRAIN CUT OF BEEF AS TERIYAKI, AND THE MARINADE IS SIMILAR. YOU NEED A VERY SHARP KNIFE.

beef with cardoons and mushrooms

1/2 cup olive oil, divided

3 pounds round steak, trimmed and cut into serving pieces

salt and pepper

2 pounds cardoons

3 anchovy fillets or 2 tablespoons fermented fish sauce

1 onion, chopped

2 cups quartered mushrooms

1/2 cup dry white wine

Heat 1/4 cup of the olive oil in a large, deep skillet with a cover. Add beef, reduce heat to simmer, and season with salt and pepper. Cover and cook for an hour. (The long cooking time makes me suspect that Abruzzians sometimes use mutton in this dish. It's a good method for my very lean, homegrown beef, but you might want to reduce the cooking time if yours is young and tender.)

Remove leaves and strings from cardoons and cut into 1-inch pieces. Cook 5 minutes in boiling water, remove from heat, and drain. In another skillet, heat remaining 1/4 cup olive oil. Add anchovies (if used), onion, and mushrooms and sauté 10 minutes.

Add vegetable mixture to beef. Stir in wine and fish sauce (if used) and cook another 5 minutes. Check seasoning and serve with polenta or rice.

Serves 6.

THIS IS INSPIRED BY A LAMB AND CARDOON DISH FROM THE ABRUZZI AND MOLISE REGIONS OF SOUTHERN ITALY. IT WAS AN INSTANT FAVORITE AT OUR HOUSE. YOU CAN SUBSTITUTE CELERY FOR ALL OR PART OF THE CARDOONS, BUT IT WON'T BE QUITE THE SAME. LAMB AND FENNEL ALSO ARE COOKED TOGETHER IN THIS STYLE.

vietnamese beef
with leeks

1 tablespoon soy sauce

1 tablespoon plus 1 teaspoon fermented fish sauce

1 teaspoon cornstarch

1/2 teaspoon honey

1 green onion, chopped, or
2 tablespoons chopped chives

1 pound rib steak, trimmed and cut into stir-fry pieces

2 tablespoons light oil

3 or 4 medium leeks, with a little green, cut into 1-inch pieces

1 tablespoon chopped cilantro (optional)

Combine soy sauce, 1 tablespoon of the fish sauce, cornstarch, honey, and green onion or chives in shallow bowl. Add beef and marinate for about an hour. Heat oil in a heavy skillet or wok. Drain meat, add to oil, and cook for 5 minutes over high heat, stirring constantly. Add leeks and the remaining teaspoon of fish sauce and cook briefly. Leeks should still be crunchy. Sprinkle with cilantro (if used) and serve hot.

Serves 4.

THE MARINADE DOES WONDERS FOR A TOUGH CUT OF BEEF. HEAVY SCISSORS
WORK MUCH BETTER THAN A KNIFE FOR TRIMMING THE FAT AND
MEMBRANE FROM AN UNDISTINGUISHED STEAK.

sooke harbour house oysters with carrot sauce

12 Pacific or golden mantle oysters, broiled or sautéed

2 medium carrots, peeled and sliced thin

1/2 small onion, sliced thin

2 cloves garlic, chopped

4 tablespoons unsalted butter, divided

2 tablespoons vermouth

1/4 cup reduced homemade fish stock

2 tablespoons lemon juice

Italian parsley or other leafy green

Melt 2 tablespoons of the butter in a saucepan, add onion and garlic, and sauté briefly. Add carrots and fish stock and cook, covered, over low heat until carrots are tender. Transfer to blender or food processor and purée. Add vermouth and lemon juice and whisk in remaining 2 tablespoons of butter. Adjust seasoning and thickness to taste.

Pour some sauce onto each of four plates. Place the oysters on the sauce—three per plate. Garnish with Italian parsley or other green and serve.

Serves 4.

GLUTEN-FREE

THIS UNUSUAL SAUCE TREATS GOOD OYSTERS WITH RESPECT, COMPLEMENTING RATHER THAN OVERWHELMING THEM. GORDON COWEN, A CHEF AT SOOKE HARBOUR HOUSE NEAR VICTORIA, BRITISH COLUMBIA, SUGGESTS SUBSTITUTING BUTTERNUT SQUASH FOR ALL OR PART OF THE CARROT FOR A VARIATION IN TASTE. GOLDEN MANTLE OYSTERS ARE RAISED IN BRITISH COLUMBIA. THEY ARE STRONGER TASTING THAN THE MORE COMMON PACIFIC OYSTER.

squid in zimino

1 tablespoon olive oil

1/2 cup chopped onion

1 clove garlic, minced

1 dried red chili pepper, minced

1/4 cup chopped parsley

1/4 cup chopped chard stem or celery

1 pound squid

1 teaspoon flour

1/2 cup dried porcini mushrooms, soaked for 30 minutes, drained and chopped, or 1 cup regular mushrooms, or a combination totaling 1 cup

1/2 cup chopped canned tomatoes

1 pound chard or beet greens

1 cup dry white wine

salt and pepper

First, clean the squid. Here's how: Grab the head and pull it from the mantle. This will bring most of the insides with it. Reach inside the mantle and remove the long piece of cartilage (called the pen) within. Rinse out the mantle. Not all recipes use the tentacles up by the head, but this one does. Chop the creature into 1/2-inch rings.

Heat olive oil in a saucepan over medium heat. Add onion, garlic, chili pepper, parsley, and chard stem or celery, reduce heat to low, and sauté until onion begins to color. Add squid and cook 10 minutes over medium heat. Sprinkle flour over top and stir it in.

Don't worry if squid is tough at this point. Add mushrooms, tomatoes, greens, and wine. Season with salt and pepper. Cover and simmer 30 minutes.

Uncover and simmer until liquid has evaporated into a coating for squid and vegetables. Serve hot, preferably over polenta.

Serves 6.

COOKING SQUID CAN BE DISCOURAGING. FIRST OF ALL, SQUID ARE UGLY, AND IF THINGS GO WRONG IN THE KITCHEN, THEY END UP CHEWY AS RUBBER BANDS. BUT WELL-COOKED SQUID ARE WONDERFUL. THE TRICK TO TENDERNESS IS EITHER TO COOK THEM VERY FAST—AS IN BLACK BEAN SAUCE CALAMARI OR FRITTO MISTO—OR FOR AT LEAST 20 MINUTES, AS IN THIS TRADITIONAL TUSCAN DISH. "IN ZIMINO" REFERS TO COOKING WITH GREENS.

black bean calamari

1 pound squid, cleaned and cut into
1/2-inch rings

1 cup carrots , julienned

1 cup celery, julienned

1/2 cup small turnips, julienned
(optional)

4 tablespoons cooking oil

1 cup black bean sauce, or more to taste

1 teaspoon black sesame seeds,
lightly toasted

1 teaspoon white sesame seeds,
lightly toasted

1/4 cup sliced green onions

Heat oil in a medium skillet until it just begins to smoke. Add carrots, celery, and turnips (if used) and toss for 30 seconds or until vegetables just begin to cook. Add squid and cook, tossing, until rings start to turn opaque, 1 minute at the most. Add black bean sauce and toss until sauce is hot, about 30 seconds. Garnish with green onions and sesame seeds.

Black bean sauce

I sometimes make a stripped-down sauce out of black beans, garlic, ginger, and soy sauce. It's good, but I admit this one is better. Fermented black beans—as well as the other seasonings for this recipe—are available in Asian markets and some supermarkets. Dry white wine can be substituted for the sake.

THIS IS FROM JOHN KEMNITZER, A FORMER SEATTLE-AREA CHEF WHO WAS A PIONEER PROMOTER OF ORGANIC AND LOCALLY SOURCED FOODS AND WHO STILL WORKS WITH REGIONAL FARMERS AND COOKS. HE DEVELOPED IT ALONG WITH RICK TADA. IT IS HEALTHFUL, AND VERY, VERY GOOD. QUICK COOKING IS THE KEY HERE, SO HAVE EVERYTHING READY IN ADVANCE. YOU CAN BUY BOTTLED BLACK BEAN SAUCE IN MOST SUPERMARKETS AS WELL AS ASIAN GROCERS. AND IF YOU ARE A STRAIGHT FROM THE WINTER GARDEN PURIST, YOU CAN SUBSTITUTE CHARD STEMS OR BLANCHED CARDOONS FOR THE CELERY.

BLACK BEAN SAUCE

1/2 cup fermented black beans

1 tablespoon minced garlic

1/2 cup low-salt soy sauce

4 teaspoons chili-garlic paste

1/2 tablespoon sesame oil

1/2 tablespoon minced fresh ginger

1/2 cup plus 3 tablespoons sake

2 tablespoons sugar

pinch of crushed red chili pepper

3/4 teaspoon ground Sichuan pepper

3/4 teaspoon Chinese five-spice powder

3 tablespoons cornstarch

3-1/2 cups water, divided

Bring 1-1/2 cups water to a boil and add black beans. Simmer 5 minutes. Strain and discard the water. Retain about a quarter of the beans for the texture and purée the rest.

Combine the remaining 2 cups water, 1/2 cup of the sake, and all remaining ingredients except cornstarch in a saucepan and bring to a boil. Add beans and return to boiling. Reduce heat to simmer. Combine cornstarch and remaining 3 tablespoons sake in a small bowl. Add slowly to black beans, whisking to mix thoroughly. Simmer gently for 5 minutes.

Serves 4 - makes 2 cups.

baked fish and chicory

2 pounds fillet of sole

2 pounds chicory

salt and pepper

1 tablespoon chopped parsley

1 large clove garlic, minced

1/2 cup olive oil

Preheat oven to 400°F.

Wash and dry sole fillets, cut lengthwise into small strips, and dry again. Tear chicory, wash, and dry carefully.

Arrange chicory and fish in alternate layers in an oiled baking dish, seasoning each layer with salt, pepper, parsley, garlic and oil. End with a layer of chicory and seasoning. Bake for 35 minutes.

Serves 6.

GLUTEN-FREE

SIMPLE PLEASURES ARE THE BEST. THE TOP LAYER OF CHICORY
WILL BROWN SLIGHTLY, BUT THAT'S FINE.

sole au vert

1 fillet of sole per diner

salt and pepper

1/4 cup flour

3 tablespoons butter, divided

1 cup chopped sorrel or spinach

2 tablespoons chopped chives

2 tablespoons chopped parsley

2 teaspoons chopped tarragon

Salt and pepper sole fillets and dust with flour. Heat 2 tablespoons of the butter in skillet and cook fillets, turning to brown lightly on both sides. Add sorrel or spinach, herbs, and the remaining 1 tablespoon butter and simmer until greens are tender but not mushy, 3 or 4 minutes.

Serves 4.

THE COMBINATION OF HERBS HERE IS A SUGGESTION, NOT AN ORDER. IF YOU DON'T USE
ANY SORREL, SPRINKLE FILLETS WITH LEMON JUICE BEFORE SERVING.

TEMPURA

Tempura is perfect for the winter garden, allowing you to combine a bit of this and a leaf of that into a harmonious meal. The ingredients must be fresh, but they need not be pretty.

Food writer Jennifer Brennan says that the Japanese acquired the technique for batter-fried food from 16th-century Portuguese traders and that the name derives from the Latin *tempora*. Russ Rudzinski, co-owner of a pioneer Japanese country-style restaurant in San Francisco, offers a Buddhist monk as an originator and a more poetic etymology: three picture characters—*tem*, meaning heaven; *pu*, meaning woman; and *ra*, meaning silken veil. Therefore, a woman veiled in silk, offering a glimpse of heaven. Anyway, it tastes great and the techniques are simple, although time-consuming and a bit messy.

Another subject of debate is the batter. Brennan emphasizes that it must be absolutely fresh, preferably made in two batches while the cooking is in progress. Rudzinski wants you to make it at least 15 minutes in advance. I'm with him, since the batter is basically the same as fritter batter, which also benefits from a refrigerated rest before cooking. I have had good results with his recipe, which I pass on here. I also have been satisfied with commercial tempura mix. However you do it, the point is to avoid activating the gluten in the flour, so that the batter doesn't get rubbery. I go into all this detail on the great tempura debate to emphasize the dangers of blindly following any expert. What works in your kitchen is the right way to do it.

You need to be attentive while frying, so prepare all the vegetables and seafood in advance.

Just one more thing: Japanese cooks also make a related dish, abura yaki, which uses the same oil but no batter. Use firm vegetables and lean meat, usually beef, all sliced about 1/4-inch thick. Fry for a few minutes in the hot oil and serve with a dipping sauce.

tempura

VEGETABLES AND SEAFOOD

broccoli florets

cauliflower florets

spinach leaves, washed and dried

sweet potatoes, peeled and sliced about 1/4-inch thick

small cubes of pumpkin or other winter squash

mushrooms, sliced lengthwise

carrots, peeled and sliced on the diagonal

celery, in 1-inch chunks

shrimp, prawns, or chunks of firm white fish

vegetable oil for frying

BATTER FOR 4

2-1/4 cups all-purpose flour, divided

1/2 teaspoon baking powder

2 eggs

2 cups ice water

Batter

Mix 2 cups of the flour with all remaining ingredients. The mixture should be the consistency of whipping cream; a few lumps are okay. Let stand 15 minutes before use.

Put remaining 1/4 cup flour in a small, shallow bowl.

Dipping Sauce

Combine all dipping ingredients and stir until sugar is dissolved.

Preparation

Shell shrimp and prawns, leaving tails attached. Clean and devein them. Score each shrimp several times across its underside to reduce curling. Butterfly large prawns open to increase cooking surface. Dry shrimp and prawns thoroughly; the batter won't stick on a wet surface.

DIPPING SAUCE

1 cup chicken stock or dashi (Japanese fish stock, available in powdered form)

1/4 cup sugar

1/2 cup soy sauce

2 tablespoons mirin or sherry

1 tablespoon grated daikon (optional)

Pour oil into a wok, deep-fat fryer, or electric frying pan. (The oil can be strained, refrigerated, and reused.) The amount of oil depends on the size of your container, but the greater the volume, the easier it is to maintain the proper temperature. Four cups is a reasonable amount for a standard wok. Heat oil to between 350°F and 375°F. If you don't have a deep-fat thermometer, test with a spoonful of batter. It should drop to the bottom of the fryer and then rise almost immediately to the surface. If the batter doesn't drop, the oil is too hot. If it doesn't rise, the oil is too cold. Starting with vegetables and ending with seafood, roll each piece in the small bowl of flour and then dip into the batter. Drain off the surplus batter, and then drop the pieces gently into the oil. Fry for 2 to 3 minutes, remove, and drain on paper towels. Do not crowd the items as they fry. They must be able to float on the surface, and the temperature must not drop below 350°F. When pieces are drained, place them on a heated serving plate and keep warm until everything is cooked. Serve immediately with small bowls of dipping sauce.

prawn curry

1/2 pound prawns

2 pounds fresh spinach or one 12-ounce box frozen spinach

3 tablespoons ghee (*see page 236*) or light oil

1 medium onion, sliced

1 clove garlic, chopped

2 inches cinnamon stick

1 teaspoon ground cumin

1/2 teaspoon turmeric

1 teaspoon ground coriander seeds

2 teaspoons chili powder

1 teaspoon black pepper

1/2 cup tomato paste

1 teaspoon honey

1 teaspoon salt

1 teaspoon garam masala (*see page 235*) or 1/2 teaspoon curry powder

Peel prawns. If spinach is fresh, chop leaves coarsely and steam for 5 minutes. Remove from heat and drain. If spinach is frozen, thaw partially and chop into 1-inch cubes. Heat oil in a large saucepan or skillet. Sauté onion and garlic until onion starts to soften. Add cinnamon, cumin, turmeric, coriander, chili powder, and black pepper. Sauté 2 minutes.

Add tomato paste and honey and cook another minute, mixing well. Add spinach and salt and stir well to coat spinach with tomato-spice mixture. Add prawns. Cook gently, turning prawns so they color on both sides. When prawns are pink, add garam masala or curry powder and cook another 5 minutes. The curry should be fairly dry, not soupy.

Serves 4.

THIS DISH IS FROM BANGLADESH. UNLIKE SOME SPICY PRAWN DISHES, IN THIS ONE YOU STILL CAN TASTE THE SEAFOOD. MINT CHUTNEY (*SEE PAGE 234*) MAKES AN EXCELLENT CONDIMENT.

moules marinière

50 mussels

1/4 cup butter

2 cloves garlic, chopped

4 tablespoons chopped shallots

3 leeks (white part only), chopped

1 bay leaf

salt and pepper

3/4 cup dry white wine

chopped parsley or cilantro

Scrub mussels and remove beards. Melt butter in soup kettle. Add garlic and shallots and cook gently for 1 minute. Add leeks and bay leaf and cook until vegetables are limp.

Add mussels, salt, pepper, and white wine. Cover and cook gently until mussels open. Discard any that don't.

Remove mussels and divide into bowls. Strain broth, return it to the kettle, and cook without boiling for 2 or 3 minutes. Pour over mussels, garnish with parsley or cilantro, and serve.

Serves 4.

GLUTEN-FREE

NOT SO MANY YEARS AGO, CLAM DIGGERS AND OYSTER GATHERERS WOULD WALK RIGHT BY SUCCULENT MUSSEL BEDS IN SEARCH OF BIGGER GAME. NOW MUSSELS ARE SO POPULAR THAT THEY ARE AVAILABLE COMMERCIALLY. WINTER IS A FINE TIME FOR THEM BECAUSE THE RED-TIDE DANGER IS AT ITS LOWEST POINT. IF YOU GATHER YOUR OWN, PICK ONLY TIGHTLY CLOSED SPECIMENS AND AVOID HIGHLY POLLUTED WATERWAYS.

CILANTRO MAKES A NICE CHANGE FROM PARSLEY IN THIS RECIPE. YOU COULD THEN CHANGE THE NAME TO MEJILLONES A LA MARINERA SO AS NOT TO OFFEND THE FRENCH.

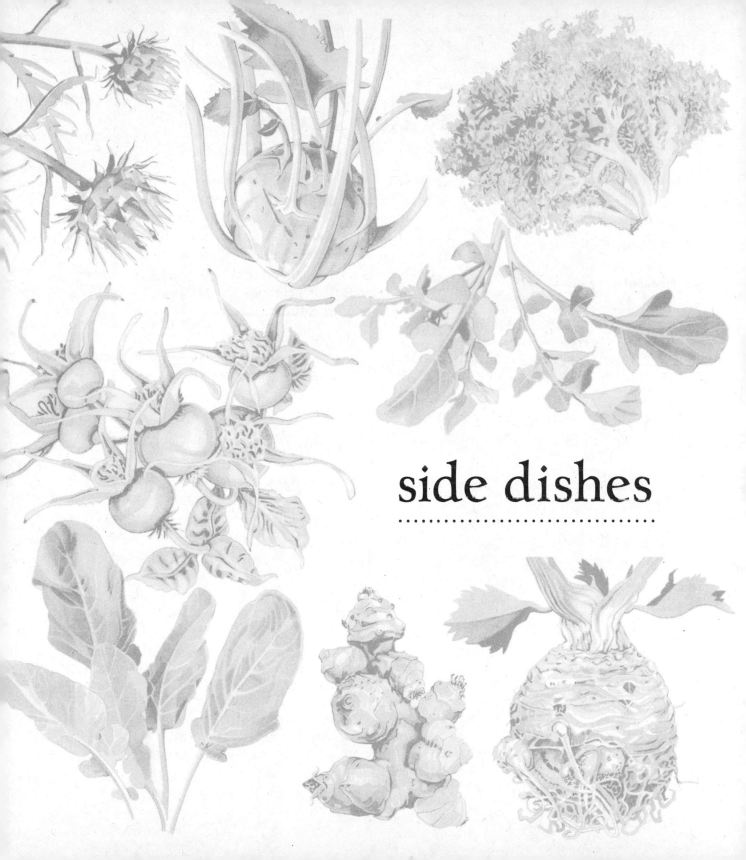

side dishes

teriyaki beets

12 small unpeeled beets

4 tablespoons butter

2 tablespoons honey

1 tablespoon finely chopped fresh ginger

1 tablespoon soy sauce

Boil or steam beets until almost tender. Time will vary with size and age of beets. Rinse in cold water, peel, and cut into halves. In a small saucepan, combine butter, honey, ginger, and soy sauce and heat until butter and honey are melted. Brush some of the sauce over beets and place on a heated broiler pan. Broil 8 or 10 minutes or until tender, basting frequently. Transfer to serving dish and pour remaining sauce over.

Serves 4 to 6.

VEGETARIAN

MANY PEOPLE THINK THEY HATE BEETS, AND I USED TO BE AMONG THEM, BUT IT'S ENTIRELY POSSIBLE THEY ONLY HATE SWEET-AND-SOUR HARVARD BEETS, WHICH ARE INDEED AN OUTRAGE. BEETS ARE NOT SUBTLE VEGETABLES, BUT THEY CAN BE DELICIOUS. THE SOY SAUCE AND GINGER IN THIS DISH ARE EXCELLENT COMPLEMENTS TO THE EARTHY SWEETNESS OF THE BEETS. YOU COULD BROIL THEM ALONGSIDE SOME NICE HALIBUT AND SERVE WITH RICE AND A GREEN SALAD.

gingered beets and brussels sprouts

1 pound Brussels sprouts (about 3 cups), trimmed

2 medium beets, boiled, baked, or steamed

2 tablespoons butter

2 teaspoons fresh grated ginger

2 tablespoons lemon juice

salt and pepper

Cut an X in the stem of each Brussels sprout and steam over boiling water until nearly tender, 5 to 7 minutes. Remove from heat. Peel and slice beets. Cut sprouts in half if they are really large. Heat butter in a medium skillet or saucepan, add sprouts, beets, and ginger, and sauté until vegetables are tender. Add lemon juice, salt, and pepper and cook very gently another 2 or 3 minutes.

Serves 4.

VEGETARIAN, GLUTEN-FREE

REALLY FRESH BRUSSELS SPROUTS ARE IMPORTANT HERE.

roasted beets

5 medium beets, either red or golden but not both together

5 tablespoons olive oil, divided

1/2 cup chopped scallions or small leeks, white part only

3/4 cup feta cheese, cubed or crumbled

1/2 cup chopped walnuts (optional)

2 tablespoons balsamic vinegar

salt and pepper

Preheat oven to 400°F.

Scrub the beets but do not peel them. Rub with a tablespoon of the olive oil and place on a silicon pad or bakers parchment on a baking dish. Roast until a knife goes all the way into the beet without much pressure and it is beginning to drip and caramelize.

Remove from oven, cool, peel and chop into 1/2 inch cubes.

Put in a serving bowl; add scallions, walnuts, and feta cheese.

Make a vinaigrette dressing with the remaining olive oil and the balsamic vinegar. Mix gently. Add salt and pepper to taste, mix again, and serve.

Serves 6 to 8.

VEGETARIAN, GLUTEN-FREE

My friend Deb and I were asked to bring vegetarian dishes to a friend's outdoor wedding. I made marinated baked tofu; she brought the most beautiful salad. Golden beets, roasted until they began to caramelize, with green onions, feta cheese, and a vinaigrette, and topped with nasturtiums. You won't find the nasturtiums in the garden in winter, but the beets and scallions are available, and the result looks romantic in any season. Red beets are fine too, but I think the golden ones are even sweeter roasted. Don't combine them. The color will bleed from the red ones and make the golden ones look mottled and strange.

It takes a long time, maybe 1-½ hours, to oven roast a good-sized beet. I used to think it made sense to cook them in the microwave, which is many times quicker, but you just don't get the same depth of flavor. So my new approach is to do a big batch at once so as not to waste the oven time. They freeze well, and should you somehow tire of the vinaigrette and feta cheese, you can alternate with skordalia sauce (*see page 228*) or a gorgonzola vinaigrette.

braised baby bok choy

1 bunch bok choy per diner

garlic

olive oil

toasted sesame oil

fresh ginger root

soy sauce

chicken stock

Preheat oven to 400°F.

Choose very small, tender baby bok choy. Slice them in two lengthwise and place them in a flat casserole, cut side down. Over them sprinkle a lot of finely chopped garlic, some olive oil, a bit of toasted sesame oil, grated fresh ginger, a splash of soy sauce and a shallow amount of good chicken stock.

Cover and place in a 400°F oven for about a half hour, uncovering for the last five to ten minutes. Save any remaining stock/juices to pour over the rice you will probably want to serve with this.

VERY EASY, VERY GOOD, AND EASILY ADAPTABLE
TO ONE DINER OR DOZENS. THE CHICKEN STOCK DOES IMPROVE THE FLAVOR,
BUT VEGANS COULD SUBSTITUTE AND STILL BE HAPPY.

broccoli romeo

broccoli or kale

garlic

salt and pepper

olive oil

Romeo Conca, who was a terrific cook, and founder of Lost Mountain Winery, which recently closed and is still missed, used this treatment to get the most flavor and nutrition out of homegrown broccoli or kale. Good cooking doesn't come any simpler than this. I quote his instructions verbatim:

"If there is no danger of cabbage worms or aphids, pick directly into a saucepan, cover the greens with water, and then drain off all the water. If there is a concern for bugs, cover with well-salted water and observe carefully. Again drain completely. The small amount of water trapped in the greens is all that's needed. Add a clove, or two if small, of garlic, some salt, a grind of pepper, and a liberal drizzle of olive oil, cover with a well-fitting lid, and cook on low heat. Depending on quantities, 10 or 15 minutes is enough. This method of cooking retains the flavor—no liquid to drain off—and so both broccoli and kale have a somewhat more pronounced flavor."

VEGAN, GLUTEN-FREE

sauté of broccoli and turnips

1 pound broccoli (about 3 cups), peeled and trimmed

3/4 pound (5 or 6) small turnips, peeled and cut into 3/4-inch wedges

2 tablespoons butter

2 tablespoons oil

1/2 teaspoon sugar

salt and pepper

Cut florets from broccoli stems. Cut stems into 1/4-inch diagonals. Steam stems 4 minutes over boiling water. Add florets and cook another 3 or 4 minutes, until barely tender. Remove broccoli and let it cool.

Put turnips in steamer and cook until barely tender, about 5 minutes. Remove from heat.

Melt butter and oil in large, heavy skillet over medium-high heat. Add turnips and sugar and stir until lightly browned. Add broccoli and toss until vegetables are heated through. Season with salt and pepper.

Serves 4.

VEGETARIAN, GLUTEN-FREE

SIMPLE AND ATTRACTIVE, THIS QUICK DISH RISES SEVERAL CULINARY NOTCHES WHEN YOU HAVE FRESH YOUNG TURNIPS. STEAM THE VEGETABLES SEPARATELY SO THAT YOU CAN MONITOR THEIR CRISPNESS CLOSELY. THEY NEED TO KEEP A LITTLE CRUNCH.

broccoli leek purée

1 bunch broccoli (about 3 cups florets)

4 or 5 medium leeks

1/2 cup cottage cheese

3 tablespoons butter

salt and pepper

freshly grated nutmeg

Steam broccoli florets over boiling water for 3 minutes. Drain, submerge in cold water, and drain again when broccoli is cool. Don't let broccoli cook until it is soft—it spoils the dish.

Trim leeks, cut into 1/2-inch pieces, and wash. Boil in salted water until tender but not mushy, about 8 minutes. Drain, rinse briefly in cold water, and press out liquid. Purée broccoli and leeks together with cottage cheese. Melt butter and add to purée. Season to taste with salt, pepper, and nutmeg.

Serves 4.

VEGETARIAN

THIS FRESH-TASTING PURÉE, FLECKED WITH LIGHT AND DARK GREEN, IS GOOD WITH ROAST POULTRY. THE SLIGHT SWEETNESS OF THE LEEKS COMPLEMENTS THE BROCCOLI, WHICH IS NOT COOKED, ONLY BLANCHED. TO MAKE IT INTO A MAIN DISH, PUT THE PURÉE INTO A CASSEROLE, PLACE SAUTÉED CHICKEN BREASTS OR SAUTÉED FISH FILLETS ON TOP, AND BAKE 10 MINUTES AT 350°F.

brussels sprouts
in lemon curry sauce

1-1/2 pounds fresh or 1 pound frozen Brussels sprouts

3 tablespoons ghee (see page 236) or light cooking oil

1 onion, sliced thin

3 cloves garlic, sliced thin

1 teaspoon ground turmeric

1-1/2 teaspoons chili powder

2 inches whole cinnamon or 1 teaspoon ground

2 teaspoons poppy seeds

1 teaspoon ground cumin

1 teaspoon ground coriander seeds

1 cup yogurt

2 tablespoons honey

juice of 1 lemon

salt and pepper

2 tablespoons chopped cilantro (optional)

Preheat oven to 400°F.

Wash and trim fresh Brussels sprouts or thaw frozen ones. Cut a slash in the base of each sprout and arrange sprouts in one layer in a large covered casserole or baking dish. Heat ghee or oil in a medium saucepan. Add onion and garlic and sauté gently until soft; don't let them burn. Add turmeric, chili powder, cinnamon, poppy seeds, and cumin and cook, stirring, for 2 to 3 minutes. Stir in ground coriander.

Transfer mixture to blender. Add yogurt, honey, and lemon juice and blend. Add salt and pepper to taste and blend again. Pour mixture over sprouts. Bake, covered, for 15 to 20 minutes. Remove cover, mix gently so that sprouts are well covered with sauce, and cook uncovered until sprouts are done, maybe another 10 minutes. Don't overcook them. Sprinkle with cilantro (if used) and serve.

Serves 4.

GLUTEN-FREE

MANY INDIAN DISHES ARE SO DISTINCTIVELY FLAVORED THAT THEY CLASH WITH ANY OTHER STYLE OF COOKING, BUT THESE CRISP SPROUTS AND THEIR TANGY SAUCE GO WELL WITH A PLAIN ROAST CHICKEN OR EVEN A MEATLOAF. YOU WILL NEED RICE TO SOAK UP THE SAUCE. FROZEN SPROUTS ARE NOT AS GOOD, BUT THEY ARE BETTER THAN REALLY TIRED FRESH ONES. YOU ALSO CAN SUBSTITUTE LIGHTLY STEAMED SLICED CABBAGE OR KOHLRABI.

brussels sprouts
in green sauce

1 pound small, firm Brussels Sprouts

6 white stalks Swiss chard

1/2 cup grated celeriac

1/2 cup water

3 tablespoons butter

1 tablespoon flour

1 cup half-and-half or unsweetened soy milk

salt and pepper to taste

nutmeg

Preheat oven to 350°F.

Boil or steam sprouts until barely tender. Drain, plunge briefly into cold water, shake off excess moisture, and transfer to a shallow buttered baking dish. Slice the chard stalks thin. Bring water to boil in a medium saucepan, add chard and celeriac and cook over medium heat until tender, about 10 minutes. Purée with cooking water, return to saucepan, and cook over low heat until reduced by half.

While chard and celeriac are reducing, melt butter in a small saucepan, sprinkle on flour, and stir over medium heat until mixture foams. Whisk in half-and-half or soy milk and continue stirring until bubbly and slightly thickened. Whisk in chard/celeriac mixture. Season with salt, pepper, and nutmeg.

Pour sauce over sprouts and toss to coat.
Bake 20 minutes.

Serves 4.

VEGETARIAN

THIS COMPANY DISH IS ONE OF JUDY GORMAN'S MANY INNOVATIVE VEGETABLE CREATIONS, WITH SOME ADJUSTMENTS FOR WINTER GARDENERS. IT IS DELICIOUS AND BEAUTIFUL, WITH BRIGHT GREEN SPROUTS PEEKING OUT OF THE PALE GREEN SAUCE. FOR A SELECTION OF HER RECIPES, CHECK OUT HER WEBSITE AT VEGETABLEGODDESS.COM.

roasted brussels sprouts and sweet potatoes

3 cups Brussels sprouts, trimmed and halved

2 cups sweet potatoes, peeled and diced

1 medium onion, roughly chopped

4 cloves garlic, peeled and sliced

3 tablespoons olive oil

salt and pepper

1 tablespoon soy sauce

a few shakes of hot sauce

Preheat oven to 400°F.

Mix all ingredients in a large bowl. Turn onto a baking dish or cookie sheets, with bakers parchment or a silicon liner. The vegetables need to be in a single layer.

Roast until sweet potatoes are soft and the Brussels sprouts still slightly firm. Stir periodically so that dried vegetables at the edge of the pan get moved into the moister center. A few browned edges are fine, in fact desired.

Serves 6 to 8.

VEGAN, GLUTEN-FREE

SEVERAL YEARS BACK I BROUGHT A ROASTED VEGETABLE DISH TO A POTLUCK—PROBABLY BRUSSELS SPROUTS, CHERRY TOMATOES, AND SWEET POTATOES—AND EVERYONE WAS CURIOUS AND COMPLIMENTARY. HOW HAD I DONE THAT? WHAT WERE THE SEASONINGS? THE IDEA WAS UNFAMILIAR. A COUPLE OF YEARS LATER, I BROUGHT THE SAME DISH TO ANOTHER POTLUCK, WHERE WE FOUND ON ASSEMBLY THAT WE HAD AMASSED FIVE COMBINATIONS OF ROASTED VEGETABLES AND NOT MUCH ELSE. CLEARLY, THE WORD WAS OUT. ROASTING VEGETABLES CONCENTRATES FLAVOR, BRINGS OUT SWEETNESS, ALLOWS FOR GREAT TASTE WITH LITTLE TO NO FAT, AND REWARDS ALL SORTS OF IMPROVISATION.

THIS IS ONE OF MY FAVORITE COMBINATIONS. THANKSGIVING REQUIRES IT AT OUR HOUSE. FOR MY DAUGHTER'S WEDDING RECEPTION, WE ADDED CHERRY TOMATOES. THAT'S OUTSIDE THE PARAMETERS OF THIS BOOK, BUT IT'S A NICE TOUCH. YOU MIGHT AS WELL MAKE A LOT; IT KEEPS SEVERAL DAYS.

cabbage with coconut

1/2 medium cabbage, sliced into thin ribbons

3 tablespoons vegetable oil

1 large onion, sliced thin

2 cloves garlic, sliced

4 hot green chilies (or fewer, according to taste), seeded and chopped

2-inch piece of fresh ginger, sliced

1 teaspoon salt

1 tablespoon unsweetened dried coconut

Steam cabbage about 5 minutes. It should still be crunchy. Remove from heat and drain. Do not dry. Heat oil in a skillet or large saucepan. Add onion, garlic, and ginger and sauté until onion begins to soften. Add chopped chilies and sauté about 2 minutes. Add cabbage, reduce heat, and mix thoroughly. Add salt and coconut and continue to cook, stirring, until coconut is moist and cabbage is heated through. It should not be completely soft. Serve warm.

Serves 4.

VEGAN, GLUTEN-FREE

A SOUTH INDIAN DISH THAT ALSO CAN BE MADE WITH SAVOY OR CHINESE CABBAGE. IT CAN BE VERY HOT, DEPENDING ON THE TYPE AND AMOUNT OF CHILIES. UNSWEETENED COCONUT IS AVAILABLE AT NATURAL FOOD STORES AND ASIAN AND INDIAN MARKETS.

stewed cardoons

4 pounds cardoons (about 8 big stalks)

3 tablespoons lemon juice

3 tablespoons olive oil

2 cups water

2 cloves garlic, sliced

2 tablespoons chopped parsley

salt and pepper

Remove any tough strings and slice cardoons into 1/2-inch pieces. Add lemon juice to a bowl of cold water, add cardoons, and let stand for 15 minutes. Drain and cook about 20 minutes in 1 inch of lightly salted water. Drain again and put in medium skillet with 2 cups water, olive oil, garlic, parsley, salt, and pepper. Cook, covered, at low heat for 30 minutes. Remove cover and continue simmering until liquid is evaporated.

Serves 6.

VEGAN, GLUTEN-FREE

THIS DISH PRESENTS THE UNADORNED FLAVOR OF CARDOONS. ONCE COOKED,
THEY CAN BE SPRINKLED WITH A CUP OF GRATED CHEESE AND RUN UNDER THE BROILER,
OR COVERED WITH CREAM SAUCE AND SOME BREAD CRUMBS AND BAKED 20 MINUTES AT 400°F.

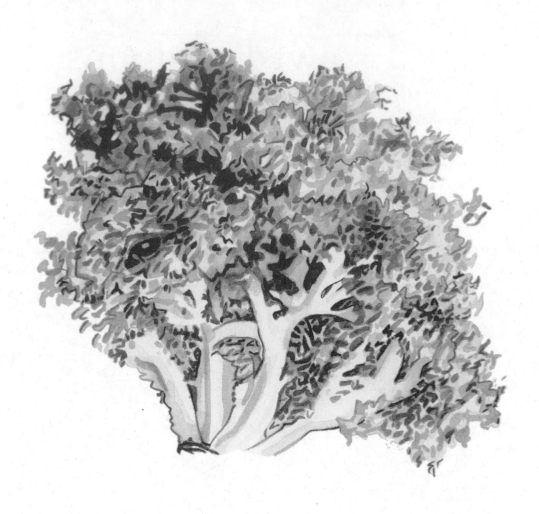

chicory

· · · · · · · · · · · · · · · ·

cardoons pellegrini

1 pound cardoons

2 ounces lean salt pork, minced and pounded to a paste

2 tablespoons olive oil

2 teaspoons butter

3 shallots or 1 small onion, minced

2 cloves garlic

1 tablespoon chopped celery leaves

1/3 cup tomato sauce

1/3 cup beef or chicken stock

3 tablespoons lemon juice

Trim and slice cardoons into 2-inch pieces and blanch 3 or 4 minutes in boiling salt water. Remove and drain. (You can save the cooking water for soup.) Melt salt pork, olive oil, and butter in a skillet. Add shallots or onion, garlic, and celery leaves and sauté gently, watching carefully so mixture does not brown. Add tomato sauce, stock, and lemon juice. Simmer a few minutes until mixture is well blended. Add cardoons, cover, and cook until tender.

Serves 4.

ANGELO PELLEGRINI TAUGHT SHAKESPEARE AT THE UNIVERSITY OF WASHINGTON, AND WROTE BOOKS INCLUDING *THE FOOD LOVER'S GARDEN* AND *THE UNPREJUDICED PALATE*, WHILE TREATING HIS LUCKY FAMILY AND FRIENDS TO ONE FEAST AFTER ANOTHER. AMONG MANY OTHER VEGETABLE CAUSES, HE CHAMPIONED CARDOONS, RAISING THEM IN HIS SEATTLE GARDEN. HE ALSO RECOMMENDED THIS RECIPE FOR USE WITH SAVOY CABBAGE, COLLARDS, KALE, AND OTHER STRONG-FLAVORED GREENS. YOU MAY NOT FEATURE SALT PORK IN YOUR DIET, AND I DON'T EITHER, USUALLY, BUT I DON'T MESS WITH PELLE'S RECIPES. THE PELLEGRINI FOUNDATION PRESENTS AN ANNUAL AWARD IN HIS HONOR, FOR THE PERSON WHO HAS BEST CARRIED ON HIS LEGACY OF THE GOOD LIFE, "AS IT ENCOMPASSES FOOD, WINE, COMMUNITY AND THE JOYS OF THE TABLE."

cardoons à la lyonnaise

1 pound slender cardoons

juice of 1 lemon, divided

2 tablespoons olive oil

1 tablespoon butter

1 tablespoon flour

1 cup vegetable stock

1 cup dry white wine

1/2 cup Gruyère cheese, grated

salt and pepper

Preheat oven to 425°F.

Cut cardoons into bite-sized pieces and sprinkle with half the lemon juice. Simmer about 30 minutes in a medium saucepan with just enough water to cover. Remove cardoons from heat, drain, and sauté in olive oil over medium heat until golden brown. Meanwhile, heat stock gently and add wine.

Melt butter in small saucepan. Add flour, stirring to mix thoroughly. Gradually add stock and wine mixture, stirring constantly. Cook gently until mixture thickens, simmer 5 more minutes, and remove from heat. Stir in cheese and remaining lemon juice.

Put cardoons in shallow casserole. Pour sauce over and bake, uncovered, 10 to 15 minutes.

Serves 4.

VEGETARIAN

YOU CAN SERVE CARDOONS WITH A SIMPLE CREAM SAUCE, BUT THE DELICATE
ARTICHOKE FLAVOR GOES ESPECIALLY WELL WITH THE BIT OF
LEMON AND GRUYÈRE IN THIS DISH.

carrots with cashews

1/2 cup light vegetable oil or ghee (*see page 236*)

1 pound carrots (3 or 4 medium), sliced on the diagonal, about 1/4-inch thick

1 large onion, sliced

2-inch piece fresh ginger, sliced thin

1 teaspoon garam masala (*see page 235*) or curry powder

1 teaspoon chili powder (omit if using curry powder)

2 teaspoons flour

1/2 pound (1-1/2 cups) cashew nuts

1/2 cup chicken or vegetable stock

salt to taste

1/2 cup canned tomatoes, seeded, drained, and chopped

Heat oil or ghee and sauté carrots and onion for 2 minutes. Add sliced ginger, garam masala, and chili powder. Cook, stirring, until vegetables are coated. Add flour and continue to stir. As mixture thickens, add cashews, stock, and salt. Bring to a boil; lower heat and simmer, covered, until carrots are tender but not mushy. Time will depend on the carrots—start checking after 10 minutes.

Add tomatoes and cook gently another 5 or 6 minutes. The sauce should be a thick coating on the carrots. If it is still very liquid, raise heat and boil briskly until excess liquid has evaporated.

Serves 4.

THIS DISH IS A GOOD CHOICE FOR NEWCOMERS TO SOUTH ASIAN COOKING,
SINCE IT IS FLAVORFUL WITHOUT BEING VERY HOT.

carrot curry

4 to 5 cups peeled and sliced carrots

1 cup fresh orange juice

1/2 cup water

1 teaspoon salt

4 tablespoons ghee (*see page 236*) or light oil

4 cardamom pods, seeded, or 1/2 teaspoon ground cardamom

1-1/2 teaspoons turmeric

1-1/2 teaspoons mustard seeds

4 cloves

1/4 teaspoon cayenne

1/2 teaspoon curry powder

1 banana, sliced thin

2 to 3 tablespoons raisins

Simmer carrots with orange juice, salt and water for about 5 minutes. Remove from heat but do not drain. Heat ghee or oil in skillet and add spices. Sauté a few minutes, using a spatula to prevent sticking. Add carrots with their liquid, raisins and banana. Simmer slowly about half an hour, until sauce is thick. Avoid unnecessary stirring so the banana slices don't disintegrate.

Serves 4 to 6.

VEGETARIAN, GLUTEN-FREE

THIS FALLS SOMEWHERE BETWEEN A CHUTNEY AND A CURRY, AND IT GOES WELL WITH INDIAN SPINACH WITH POTATOES (*SEE PAGE 126*). THE SPICES KEEP THE CARROTS AND FRUIT FROM BEING INSIPIDLY SWEET.

georgian-style cauliflower

1 small cauliflower, separated into florets

4 tablespoons butter or light oil, divided

2 small onions, finely chopped

4 tablespoons minced parsley

2 tablespoons minced cilantro

2 large eggs, beaten

salt and pepper

Steam cauliflower over boiling water for 10 minutes. Remove from heat and drain. Meanwhile, sauté onions in a large pan with 3 tablespoons of the butter or oil until golden. Add the remaining 1 tablespoon of butter or oil and stir in cauliflower, turning florets to coat them well. Cook, covered, for 10 minutes more, until tender.

Stir in parsley, cilantro, and eggs. Toss mixture gently to distribute the egg coating and then cook only until the eggs are done. Season to taste.

Serves 4.

VEGETARIAN, GLUTEN-FREE

CAULIFLOWER AND CILANTRO ARE AN EXCELLENT COMBINATION, OFTEN FOUND IN CURRIES. THIS DISH FROM GEORGIA (THE COUNTRY, NOT THE STATE) USES THE SAME FLAVORS TO DIFFERENT EFFECT, ACCENTUATING THE SWEETNESS OF A REALLY FRESH CAULIFLOWER.

celeriac and potatoes

2-1/2 to 3 pounds celeriac (about 4 medium roots), peeled and cut into 1/2-inch slices

2 cups warm mashed potatoes

3 to 4 tablespoons butter, divided

1/2 teaspoon salt

pepper

Put celeriac in saucepan with 2 tablespoons butter, salt, and enough water to barely cover. Bring to boil, cover, and simmer slowly for 25 to 30 minutes or until tender. Uncover and cook until any liquid evaporates.

Purée celeriac and combine with potatoes. Warm briefly, season with pepper to taste, and stir in the remaining butter.

Another classic recipe omits the potatoes and uses 3/4 pound of apples to each pound of celeriac. Cook the celeriac for 20 minutes before adding the peeled, sliced apples. When the apples are tender, purée the mixture. Add milk or cream until you reach the consistency you want, season with salt and pepper to taste, and serve.

Serves 8.

VEGETARIAN, GLUTEN-FREE

CELERIAC PURÉES WELL, AND ITS MILD, SLIGHTLY SWEET FLAVOR COMBINES NICELY WITH OTHER VEGETABLES. EXPERIMENTATION WILL SHOW YOU WHICH COMBINATIONS YOUR FAMILY LIKES BEST. POTATOES ARE ALWAYS A GOOD PLACE TO START.

celeriac and cheese

4 medium celeriacs, peeled

2 large eggs, separated

1/2 cup whole milk or half-and-half

salt and pepper

1 cup grated Gruyère or other firm cheese

1 cup plain yogurt

3 tablespoons lemon juice

1 tablespoon chopped fresh parsley

Cook celeriacs in boiling water until tender, about 30 minutes. Drain. Cut into quarters and purée, using as much of the milk or half-and-half as necessary to get the mixture smooth.

Preheat oven to 350°F.

Combine purée, egg yolks, remaining milk, salt, and pepper in a mixing bowl. Beat until well blended and stir in cheese. Beat egg whites into soft peaks and fold into the celeriac mixture.

Pour into a large buttered casserole or a 5-by-9-inch loaf pan. There must be enough room for the mixture to rise. Cover and bake until a tester comes out clean, about 30 to 40 minutes.

Allow to cool for 5 minutes and unmold onto a serving plate. Serve with a sauce made of the yogurt, lemon juice, and parsley.

Serves 6 as a side dish or 4 as a main dish.

VEGETARIAN, GLUTEN-FREE

bagna cauda

1 cup olive oil

4 tablespoons butter

3 teaspoons finely chopped garlic

10 to 12 anchovy fillets (one small can), chopped fine

fresh raw vegetables suitable for dipping, such as broccoli, sliced carrots, radishes, spinach leaves, young kale, kohlrabi, celeriac and blanched cardoons

Heat oil and butter until mixture foams slightly. Add garlic and sauté over low heat for about 3 minutes. Add anchovies and cook gently until they dissolve into a paste. Keep sauce hot at the table and stir occasionally to keep the anchovies blended. Provide lots of bread for dipping.

Serves 4.

Bagna Cauda ("hot bath") is a traditional northern Italian winter dish, featuring the small, sweet cardoons of the Piedmont region and other cold weather roots and greens. It's similar in concept to the Japanese abura yaki (*see page 147*), although the vegetables are simmered rather than fried, and to fondue, right across the border in Switzerland. The vegetables and sauce can be prepared ahead of time, allowing instant gratification after a day out in the cold. Keep cardoon slices in acidulated water until serving time so they don't turn brown. Use a candle warmer or a fondue set-up to keep the sauce hot at the table. Serve with excellent bread.

braised daikon

1-1/2 pounds fresh daikon, peeled and diced

2 tablespoons light cooking oil

1 teaspoon sugar

1-1/2 tablespoons soy sauce

1/4 cup water

Put daikon in a saucepan, cover with water, and bring to a boil. Boil for about 5 minutes, drain, and set aside. Heat a skillet or heavy saucepan, add oil, and stir-fry daikon for 2 minutes. Add sugar and soy sauce. Stir and mix for another minute so that sugar and soy coat daikon. Add water, cover, and bring to boil. Reduce heat to medium-low and cook about 30 minutes or until daikon is tender but not mushy. Stir occasionally to keep daikon coated with sauce. Serve hot.

Serves 4.

VEGAN

THE SIMPLE SAUCE CARAMELIZES SLIGHTLY, AND THE RESULTING DISH
IS VERY APPEALING. IT GOES WELL WITH A ROAST,
WITH BAKED FISH, OR WITH JAPANESE DISHES.

ethiopian collards and cottage cheese

SPICED CHEESE

12 ounces cottage cheese

1/3 cup niter kibbeh (*see page 231*)

2 garlic cloves, slightly crushed,
not chopped

1/4 teaspoon ground cardamom

1/2 teaspoon salt

1/4 teaspoon pepper

GREENS

2 pounds collards, chopped,
with stems removed

2 tablespoons minced chili pepper

1 tablespoon fresh grated ginger

1 teaspoon minced garlic

1/2 teaspoon ground cardamom

2 teaspoons minced onion

1/4 cup niter kibbeh

⊰ cook's note

Ethiopian cottage cheese is tarter and drier than the standard North American type and is closer to my homemade version. Some groceries sell dry cottage cheese, which is similar. Increase the amount of niter kibbeh in the cheese part of the recipe if you are using dry cottage cheese.

Mix cottage cheese, the 1/3 cup of niter kibbeh, garlic, cardamom, salt, and pepper together and let flavors combine at room temperature for 15 minutes.

Steam collards for about 20 minutes (less if the leaves are young and tender). Put collards in a bowl. Add chili pepper, ginger, garlic, cardamom, onion, and the 1/4 cup of niter kibbeh and mix thoroughly. Remove garlic from cottage cheese. Serve collards and cheese in separate dishes, or spoon greens over the cheese in one large bowl.

Serves 6 to 8.

VEGETARIAN, GLUTEN-FREE

NITER KIBBEH, A SPICED CLARIFIED BUTTER, GIVES THIS DISH ITS UNIQUE FLAVOR.
I HAD NEVER IMAGINED COLLARDS COULD TASTE SO GOOD.

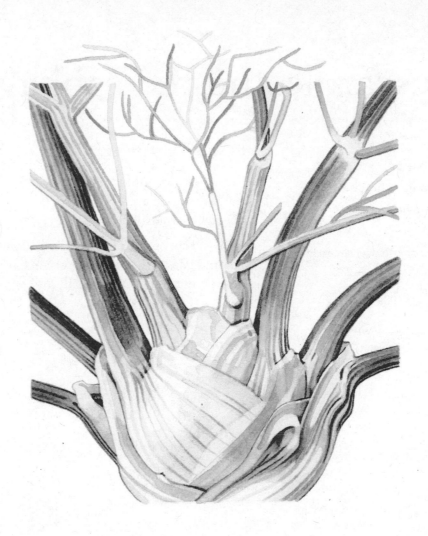

florence fennel

escarole and red cabbage

2 tablespoons vegetable oil

2 tablespoons butter

1 head red cabbage, shredded

2 teaspoons caraway seed

1 cup water

1 head escarole or chicory, sliced into shreds

salt and pepper

Heat oil and butter in a large skillet. Add cabbage and toss to coat. Cook, stirring, over medium heat for 1 minute. Add caraway seed, pour in water, and reduce heat. Cover pan and simmer for 10 to 12 minutes or until cabbage is almost tender.

Add escarole or chicory and stir to combine. Increase heat and cook, stirring, until greens are limp and liquid is evaporated. Season with salt and pepper.

Serves 6.

VEGETARIAN, GLUTEN-FREE

THE RED-VIOLET CABBAGE AND BRIGHT GREEN ESCAROLE MAKE THIS AN EXCEPTIONALLY BEAUTIFUL DISH, PROVIDED YOU SERVE IT RIGHT AWAY. IT TASTES EVEN BETTER THE NEXT DAY, BUT THE COLOR CHANGES TO A UNIFORM AND PECULIAR PURPLE. THE SMOOTH LEAVES OF ESCAROLE CONTRAST NICELY WITH THE CABBAGE, BUT THE DISH ALSO CAN BE MADE WITH CHICORY.

simplest braised fennel

fennel bulbs, sliced thick

1 tablespoon olive oil per bulb

1 garlic clove per bulb, bruised

salt

1/3 cup water per bulb

pepper

chopped fennel leaves, for garnish

Heat olive oil in a heavy skillet or saucepan. Add garlic and cook briefly over medium heat. Add lightly salted fennel slices and cook about 10 minutes at medium-low.

Add water, scrape bottom of pan, cover, and cook gently about 20 minutes. Serve with a sprinkling of pepper and chopped fennel leaves.

2 medium bulbs serve 4.

VEGAN, GLUTEN-FREE

BRAISING IN A LITTLE WATER CONCENTRATES THE FLAVOR OF THE FENNEL.
THIS SIMPLE DISH IS GOOD WITH BROILED FISH OR PORK.

simmered fennel

3 large fennel bulbs

2 tablespoons olive oil

2 cloves garlic, chopped fine

1 medium onion, chopped fine

1/2 cup vegetable broth, divided

1/2 cup dry white wine

1/2 cup cooked rice (optional)

2 tablespoons tomato sauce

salt and pepper

Trim fennel, cut into medium wedges, and set aside. Heat oil in a large saucepan. Add garlic and onion and sauté over medium heat until they begin to color, about 5 minutes. Add fennel, 1/4 cup of the broth, wine, tomato sauce, rice (if used), and salt and pepper.

Cover and cook over low heat, stirring occasionally, until fennel is tender, about 20 minutes. Add broth as necessary to prevent sticking. The mixture should be moist but not swimming. Serve hot.

Serves 4 to 6.

VEGAN

FENNEL'S LICORICE FLAVOR IS SOMEWHAT MUTED HERE.

kimpira gobo:
stir-fried burdock

1-1/2 pounds gobo

2 tablespoons oil, divided

1/3 to 1/2 cup soy sauce

2 teaspoons sugar

1/4 cup dried shrimp (optional)

1/2-inch piece of fresh chili pepper, chopped, or 1/4 teaspoon dried red pepper flakes

Scrub gobo, peel, and slice into 2-inch matchsticks. Soak for 20 minutes in cold water. Mix 1 tablespoon of the oil, soy sauce, and sugar in a small bowl. Heat remaining tablespoon of oil in a medium skillet, add shrimp (if used), and sauté briefly over medium-high heat. Drain gobo, add to skillet, and cook 2 or 3 minutes. Add sauce and cook, stirring often, until most of the liquid is absorbed. Gobo should still be crisp. Add chili pepper or pepper flakes and serve.

Serves 4.

I GOT THIS RECIPE FROM MY DEAR FRIEND DEB ANDERSON-FREY, WHO GOT IT FROM HER GRANDMOTHER IN HAWAII. IT GOES WONDERFULLY WITH FRIED TOFU AND OTHER MILD DISHES. PEELING THE SLENDER, WIGGLY BURDOCK ROOTS IS A BIT FRUSTRATING, BUT EVERYTHING ELSE IS EASY. DRIED SHRIMP ARE AVAILABLE IN ASIAN MARKETS. YOU ARE SUPPOSED TO SOAK THEM FIRST, BUT I LIKE THE TEXTURE WHEN THEY ARE ADDED TO THIS DISH DRY.

garbanzo beans with greens

3 tablespoons olive oil

1 tablespoon butter

1 garlic clove, minced or pressed

1 head escarole, cut across in 1/2-inch slices

1 teaspoon grated lemon peel (optional)

1/4 cup chopped parsley

salt and pepper

1 cup cooked garbanzo beans, drained

2 tablespoons lemon juice

Heat oil and butter in a large skillet until butter is melted. Add garlic and stir briefly over medium heat. Don't let it brown. Immediately add escarole to skillet and continue stirring over medium heat until it is wilted. Add lemon peel (if used) and parsley. Season with salt and pepper and mix in garbanzos. Stir gently over medium heat until beans are warmed through. Transfer to a serving bowl, sprinkle on lemon juice, and serve immediately.

Serves 6.

GLUTEN-FREE, VEGETARIAN

BRIEF COOKING GIVES THIS QUICK DISH A FRESH TASTE. IT ALSO CAN BE SERVED CHILLED.

adobo greens

2 pounds fresh greens

3 cloves garlic, minced

1/3 cup oil

1 tablespoon lemon or lime juice

3 tablespoons soy sauce

1/2 teaspoon salt

pepper

Chop greens roughly. Cut small stems into bite-sized pieces; discard large ones. Heat oil in a large skillet, add garlic, and sauté until it turns golden. Add greens, sauté briefly, and then add lemon or lime juice, soy sauce, and salt. Cover and bring to a boil. Remove from heat, add pepper, and serve immediately.

Serves 4.

VEGAN

ADOBO IS PROBABLY THE BEST-KNOWN TYPE OF FILIPINO COOKING.
USUALLY IT FEATURES CHICKEN, PORK, OR A COMBINATION OF THE TWO, FIRST MARINATED
IN A VINEGAR/SOY SAUCE, THEN BOILED, THEN FRIED. A SIMILAR TREATMENT WORKS
WELL WITH GREENS, WITH LEMON OR LIME JUICE SUBSTITUTED FOR VINEGAR.
TRY THIS WITH SPINACH, YOUNG CHARD, OR MILD MUSTARD GREENS.

southern mixed greens

3 pounds sturdy greens—collards, kale, beet greens, chard—coarsely chopped

2 ham hocks

1 quart water

1 teaspoon red pepper flakes

1 medium onion, chopped fine

2 tablespoons red wine vinegar

pepper

Trim excess fat from ham hocks and set it aside. Put ham hocks in a heavy saucepan or stove-top casserole. Cover with water, add red pepper flakes, and bring to a boil. Lower heat and simmer about 45 minutes.

Render some of the pork fat in a skillet. Add onions and cook slowly until they are soft and beginning to brown. Drain onions and add to ham-hock broth. Simmer another half hour or until meat begins to fall from bones.

Remove meat, trim off visible fat, and return meat to the pot. Stir in greens. Cover pot closely and cook about half an hour, stirring and lifting the greens occasionally.

Add vinegar and pepper to taste. The ham hocks should provide enough salt. Put meat and greens on a serving plate and serve pot liquor in separate small bowls. You'll want rice, biscuits, or cornbread to sop up the juice.

Serves 4.

MEALS LIKE THESE TURNED SUBSISTENCE—FORAGED GREENS AND SCRAPS FROM THE BUTCHERED HOG—INTO SOMETHING MUCH BETTER THAN JUST SURVIVAL. SLICED ORANGES MAKE A NICE ACCOMPANIMENT, AND THEY MAKE ME FEEL BETTER ABOUT THE VITAMIN C THAT HAS BEEN COOKED OUT OF THE GREENS. IF YOU WANT TO THROW ALL CHOLESTEROL CAUTION TO THE WINDS, COOK THE ONIONS WITH A QUARTER POUND OF BACON AND ADD THE COOKED BACON TO THE POT.

hortopita

1 pound mixed greens (I've used spinach, chard, romaine lettuce, rocket, nettles, sorrel, young beet greens, and turnip greens)

1/4 cup olive oil

1/2 cup finely chopped leek or onion

6 sprigs mint, chopped

1/2 cup chopped parsley

4 tablespoons cooked rice

1/2 pound filo dough, or pastry for double-crust pie

1/4 cup melted butter (if using filo dough)

Clean and stem greens. Steam leaves until limp, rinse in cold water, press out excess moisture, and chop fine. (If you have a great range of textures—say new sorrel and tough old chard—steam the vegetables separately.) Heat olive oil in a heavy skillet. Add onion or leek and cook until soft. Add chopped greens, mint, and parsley and sauté for a few minutes. Stir in rice and cook until mixture is amalgamated. It should be fairly dry.

If using filo, pick up one sheet and place it gently in a shallow casserole or baking dish. Brush lightly with melted butter and repeat with half the filo. Skip the butter if you are using pie pastry. Spread filling over pastry and top with the rest of the buttered filo or the rest of the pastry. With a sharp knife, trim excess dough from around the edges. If using filo, bake 30 minutes at 350°F. If using pie pastry, start with 10 minutes at 425°F and then reduce to 350°F for another 20 minutes.

Serves 4 to 6.

VEGETARIAN

THIS GREEK RECIPE IS A COUNTRY COUSIN OF THE RICHER SPANAKOPITA, WHICH INVOLVES EGGS AND FETA CHEESE ALONG WITH SPINACH. I LIKE TO MAKE IT IN FEBRUARY OR MARCH, WHEN MY OVERWINTERED GREENS ARE STAGING A COMEBACK AND THE FIRST WILD GREENS ARE UP. IT SHOULD BE MADE WITH FILO DOUGH, BUT IN A PINCH IT'S GOOD WITH A LIGHT DOUBLE PIE CRUST. A GREAT POTLUCK DISH.

soy sauce vegetables

2 cups any firm vegetables—turnips,
daikon, kohlrabi, carrots, beets,
and so on

1/2 teaspoon salt

2 teaspoons sugar

mild soy sauce

Cut vegetables along the grain into julienne strips.
Put them in a large jar with a lid. Add salt and sugar
and shake well so that vegetables are coated. Let
stand at room temperature for at least an hour
or up to overnight.

Pour in enough soy sauce to cover vegetables. Press
down to get rid of air pockets and let stand at room
temperature for a day. Drain off soy sauce. (It can
be reused for pickling or cooking.)

The vegetables will keep indefinitely in the refrigerator.

Makes 2 cups.

VEGAN

THIS RESEMBLES THE LITTLE PICKLED SIDE DISHES SERVED AT JAPANESE CAFÉS.
I LIKE IT BEST WITH TURNIPS AND DAIKON.

jerusalem artichokes
with rice

4 tablespoons olive oil

1 small carrot, peeled and sliced thin

1 small onion, chopped

3 cups (about 1 pound) Jerusalem artichokes, scrubbed and cut into 1/2 inch cubes

juice of 1 lemon

salt and pepper

2 tablespoons long-grain rice

1/2 cup water

2 tablespoons chopped parsley

Heat oil in large, shallow saucepan or skillet. Add carrot and onion and sauté over medium heat for 5 minutes, until vegetables begin to soften. Add Jerusalem artichokes and cook another 2 minutes, stirring constantly. Add lemon juice, salt, pepper, rice, and water. Simmer, covered, until artichokes are tender and rice is soft, about 20 minutes. Add water as necessary, a little at a time, during cooking, but do not stir. The dish should be moist but not soupy. Serve at room temperature.

Serves 4.

THE ORIGINAL OF THIS TURKISH DISH HAS A RATHER INDIGESTIBLE NAME, ZEYTINYAĞLI YER ELMASIYRA. IT IS A SORT OF RISOTTO, WITH THE SAME MOIST TEXTURE AS ITS ITALIAN COUNTERPARTS. GENTLE-FLAVORED AND RATHER SWEET, IT IS A GOOD COMPANION TO A ROAST AND A MIXED GREEN SALAD.

earth apples in olive oil

3/4 cup chopped onion

1/4 cup olive oil

1-1/2 pounds Jerusalem artichokes, cut in one-inch cubes (*see note below*)

2 tablespoons uncooked white rice

1-1/2 cups water

1/4 teaspoon salt

Italian parsley

lemon juice

lemon wedges

Sauté onions in olive oil until soft. Add artichokes and sauté another few minutes. Add rice to water, and a pinch of salt. Cover and simmer until vegetables are tender. Start checking after 20 minutes; the chokes should be barely tender. Add more salt and lemon juice to taste. Can be made up to 3 days in advance and kept refrigerated. Serve at room temperature, with lemon wedges.

Serves 4.

VEGAN, GLUTEN-FREE

THIS WAS DESIGNED FOR THE SMOOTH-SKINNED TURKISH VERSION OF THE JERUSALEM ARTICHOKE, KNOWN TO TURKS AS EARTH APPLES. THE CLOSEST APPROXIMATION I'VE FOUND IS THE RED FUSEAU VARIETY (SEE VEGETABLE LIST). THEY DON'T NEED PEELING. IF YOU ARE USING THE LUMPIER STAMPEDE TYPE, PEELING MAY BE MORE EFFECTIVE THAN TRYING TO SCRUB DIRT OUT OF EVERY LITTLE KNOB AND CREVICE.

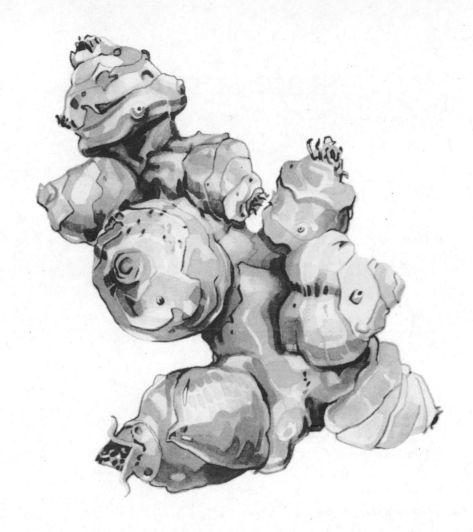

jerusalem artichoke

kale sprouts

kale buds

When the flower buds start forming on your kale plants in the spring, pick stalks that are about half as long as asparagus. Cut off any tough parts and stick the bottoms of the stalks in a small, deep pan so the buds are at the top. Add a little water and boil, covered, for no more than 5 minutes. The tougher stalks boil, and the tender buds steam.

Serve with lemon and butter.

A KALE-AND-FAREWELL SUGGESTION FOR GARDENERS,
FROM MY FRIEND BINDA COLEBROOK.

baked kohlrabi and fennel

1 fennel bulb

2 cups peeled kohlrabi, sliced about 1/2-inch thick

2 cups light soup stock (beef, chicken, or vegetable)

3 tablespoons butter, divided

2 tablespoons flour

salt and pepper

2/3 cup milk or half-and-half

1/4 cup grated Parmesan cheese

1/2 teaspoon paprika

Preheat oven to 350°F.

Strip stringy outer leaves of fennel. Slice the bulb to match kohlrabi. Bring stock to a boil, add vegetables, and cook until tender, about 7 to 10 minutes. Add enough stock to the milk or half-and-half to total 2 cups. Make a white sauce using 2 tablespoons of the butter, the flour, and the milk/stock mixture. Butter a casserole dish with remaining 1 tablespoon of butter and put in vegetables. Pour sauce over them, sprinkle with Parmesan cheese and paprika, and bake for about half an hour.

Serves 4 to 6.

A LIGHT SAUCE BRINGS OUT THE DELICATE FLAVORS OF KOHLRABI AND FENNEL.

leeks with lime

2 cloves garlic

6 medium leeks, washed and trimmed

1 cup water

1/2 teaspoon saffron (optional)

1 teaspoon salt

2-inch stalk cinnamon

2 bay leaves

2 teaspoons olive oil

1/2 teaspoon black pepper

1/2 teaspoon chili powder

1/2 teaspoon mace

juice of 6 limes or 3 large lemons

Peel and crush garlic and rub cloves over leeks. Reserve garlic for marinade. Simmer leeks, water, saffron (if used), salt, cinnamon, and bay leaves for 15 minutes. Remove leeks from pan and return liquid to heat. Boil gently until reduced by half. Remove from heat and cool. Discard cinnamon stick and bay leaves. Beat in olive oil, pepper, chili powder, and mace. Add reserved garlic and lime or lemon juice, pour over leeks, and marinate at least 2 hours.

Serves 4.

VEGAN, GLUTEN-FREE

AN INTERESTING INDIAN VARIATION ON LEEKS VINAIGRETTE.
COOKING TIME WILL VARY WITH THE SIZE AND FIRMNESS OF YOUR LEEKS.
THEY SHOULD END UP TENDER BUT NOT MUCILAGINOUS.

stir-fried leeks and romaine

1/4 cup water

2 tablespoons soy sauce

2 tablespoons rice vinegar or raspberry vinegar

3 tablespoons vegetable oil

4 medium leeks, white and light green, cut in half lengthwise and sliced very thin

1 medium head romaine, shredded

1 teaspoon red pepper flakes

Combine water, soy sauce, and vinegar in a small bowl and set aside. Heat oil in wok or large skillet. Add leeks, tossing to coat evenly. Stir over high heat for 30 seconds. Add romaine and toss to combine.

Pour on soy mixture and reduce heat. Sprinkle with red pepper flakes. Continue stirring over medium heat until all the liquid is evaporated. Serve at once.

Serves 4.

VEGAN

ROMAINE MAKES A FINE STIR-FRY GREEN. DON'T TURN YOUR BACK ON IT, THOUGH—IT COOKS ALMOST INSTANTLY. RICE VINEGAR IS STANDARD FOR THIS SAUCE, BUT I LIKE IT WITH RASPBERRY VINEGAR.

basque leeks

12 medium leeks

1 tablespoon olive oil or unsalted butter

salt and pepper

Position broiler rack 4 inches from heat source and preheat.

Trim all but 1 inch of green from leeks. Remove any tough outer leaves. Beginning about 1 inch from the base, split leeks upward, using a sharp, thin knife.

Wash leeks thoroughly, drain, and pat dry. Arrange on a large sheet of heavy aluminum foil. Rub each leek with olive oil or dot with butter. Sprinkle with salt and pepper to taste. Enclose completely in foil, wrapping tightly. Transfer to broiler pan or baking sheet. Broil 5 minutes on each side. Serve immediately.

Serves 6.

VEGAN, GLUTEN-FREE

These can go next to the salmon in the last outdoor grilling of the season or under the broiler indoors. Leeks can also be trimmed, washed, steamed lightly, and then briefly broiled without the foil wrapping. Sprinkle with salt and pepper and brush with olive oil as they cook.

saffron leeks and potatoes

3 tablespoons olive oil

3 garlic cloves, sliced

3 large leeks, trimmed, with some green,
cut into 3-inch strips

1/2 cup tomato sauce

pinch of saffron, crumbled and soaked
in a little water

salt and pepper

1 pound potatoes (3 medium), peeled
and sliced into 1/2-inch rounds

2 tablespoons chopped parsley

Heat oil in a large skillet or shallow saucepan, add
garlic, and sauté for 2 minutes. Add leeks, tomato sauce,
saffron and its soaking water, salt, pepper, and enough
water to barely cover vegetables. Simmer, covered,
10 minutes. Add potatoes and parsley. Mix well, cover,
and simmer until the potatoes are tender and water is
absorbed, about 15 minutes. Serve hot.

Serves 4.

VEGAN

THIS SPANISH COMBINATION IS ADDICTIVE. MY ONLY COMPLAINT IS THAT
I NEVER HAVE LEFTOVERS. IT MAKES A GOOD MAIN DISH AS LONG AS YOU
HAVE A BIT MORE PROTEIN ELSEWHERE IN THE MEAL.

leeks in poor man's sauce

12 medium leeks, with 2 inches of green

1 cup Poor Man's Sauce (*see recipe below*)

2 hard-boiled eggs, sieved or chopped fine

1/2 teaspoon dried tarragon

2 tablespoons chopped parsley

POOR MAN'S SAUCE

4 green onions or small leeks, minced

2 tablespoons chopped parsley

2 shallots, minced, or 1 tablespoon finely chopped onion

3 tablespoons red wine vinegar

1/2 cup olive oil

salt and pepper

Trim leeks and cut in half lengthwise. Steam until tender, remove from heat, and cool. Mix Poor Man's Sauce with eggs, tarragon, and parsley and pour over leeks. Chill at least 1 hour.

Poor Man's Sauce

Put all ingredients in a jar with a tight lid. Shake well.

Serves 4.

VEGETARIAN

POOR MAN'S SAUCE IS A VERY OLD RECIPE, A STRONGLY FLAVORED VINAIGRETTE.
IT'S GOOD ON A VARIETY OF COLD COOKED VEGETABLES, INCLUDING CARROTS,
BROCCOLI, AND JERUSALEM ARTICHOKES.

winter squash with onions

2/3 cup flour

salt and pepper

2 cups cubed winter squash

3 cups diced yellow onions

1 teaspoon dried thyme

olive oil

Put the flour, salt and pepper in a large mixing bowl (or you can do what my mom did when flouring stew meat and put it in a paper bag). Add the squash and onions and coat evenly, by tossing the veggies in the bowl or shaking the bag.

Heat 1/2 inch of olive oil in a large, heavy skillet. Watch it carefully and don't let it smoke. Olive oil has a lower smoking point than many frying oils, but you want it for the flavor. Use a slotted spoon (to remove extra flour) to add the vegetables in two or three batches, depending on the size of the pan. They need enough room to fry rather than steam from the moisture in the onions.

Fry until browned on one side and then turn over and brown the other side, maybe 4 minutes per side. Remove from heat and drain. Repeat with the remaining squash and onions.

Sprinkle with thyme, check for more salt and pepper if needed, and serve hot.

Serves 4.

VEGAN

NOVEMBER 26 IS INTERNATIONAL ONION DAY, WHICH IS THE KIND OF HOLIDAY I CAN GET BEHIND. IT'S ALSO MY SON-IN-LAW RONNY'S BIRTHDAY, ANOTHER BIG DAY AROUND HERE. I'M VERY FOND OF BOTH—RONNY AND ONIONS. THIS GREEK RECIPE REMINDS ME OF GOOD DINER FOOD—MAYBE THOSE SWEET POTATO FRIES THAT EVEN THE HEALTHIEST EATER CAN'T RESIST EVERY NOW AND THEN.

whole grain pasta with onion sauce

5 tablespoons olive oil, divided

2 pounds of onions (about three medium), sliced thin

1/2 teaspoon red pepper flakes, or more to taste

salt and pepper

1/4 cup chopped parsley

1/2 cup grated Parmesan cheese

1 pound whole grain pasta

Heat 3 tablespoons of the olive oil in a large skillet, add onions and red pepper flakes, cover, and cook over low heat for 15 minutes, stirring occasionally. Remove cover, raise heat to medium, and cook until onions brown, about 10 minutes more. Add salt, pepper, parsley, remaining 2 tablespoons of olive oil, and Parmesan cheese. Set aside.

Meanwhile, bring 4 quarts salted water to a boil, add pasta, and cook, uncovered, until pasta is al dente. Drain pasta, mix with sauce, and serve immediately. Pass more Parmesan cheese.

Serves 6.

VEGETARIAN

I'VE NEVER BEEN ENTIRELY HAPPY WITH WHOLE WHEAT PASTA, MUCH AS I APPROVE OF THE IDEA. SOMETHING ABOUT THE GRITTY TEXTURE JUST DOESN'T SEEM RIGHT WITH MOST SAUCES. HOWEVER, THEIR VARIETY IS INCREASING, THE QUALITY IS IMPROVING, AND THE RIGHT SAUCE CAN MAKE A BIG DIFFERENCE. UNLIKE MORE REFINED PASTA DISHES, WHERE THE SAUCE PROVIDES TEXTURAL INTEREST AS WELL AS FLAVOR, WHAT YOU WANT WITH WHOLE WHEAT IS SOMETHING WITH PLENTY OF TASTE BUT A SMOOTH FEEL. THIS SLOW-COOKED ONION MIXTURE IS JUST RIGHT. MIX WITH A FEW ANCHOVIES, AND YOU'VE GOT AN EXCELLENT PIZZA TOPPING.

cider-glazed parsnips

4 medium parsnips

2 tablespoons butter

1/4 cup fresh sweet cider

salt and pepper

1/4 teaspoon freshly grated nutmeg

Wash and peel parsnips and cook in lightly salted boiling water for about 10 minutes. Drain and slice, discarding any woody core.

Melt butter in frying pan and add cider. Bring to a boil, add parsnips, and cook uncovered at medium heat until liquid has evaporated and parsnips are beginning to color. Sprinkle with nutmeg.

Serves 6.

VEGETARIAN, GLUTEN-FREE

THE QUALITY OF THE CIDER MAKES A DIFFERENCE HERE. IF YOU CAN, SPLURGE ON UNFILTERED, UNRECONSTITUTED, LOCALLY PRODUCED CIDER.

simplest parsnips

small, fresh parsnips—still firm and no bigger than a large carrot

olive oil

salt

Preheat oven to 425°F.

Scrub but don't peel the parsnips. You can cut off the long skinny root ends if they are unaesthetic.

Roll them in olive oil and sprinkle with salt.

Roast until beginning to brown on the outside and soft on the inside. Start checking after 20 minutes. Serve hot and eat with your fingers.

Once you've established the baseline taste, you may want to experiment with the seasonings: spicy rubs, garlic salt, soy sauce, whatever your cupboards and menu suggest.

VEGAN, GLUTEN-FREE

SIMPLE, BUT NOT BORING. THIS TREATMENT ADDS A TOUCH OF CONTRAST AND INTEREST TO THE OFTEN-BLAND SWEETNESS OF THE ROOT. PREP TIME IS ABOUT 90 SECONDS.

english parsnip pie

2 pounds parsnips

1 teaspoon salt

2 tablespoons honey

pinch of ginger

1/4 teaspoon cinnamon

1 tablespoon fresh orange juice

2 teaspoons grated fresh orange rind
(optional)

2 eggs, slightly beaten

pastry for single-crust 9-inch pie,
partially baked, with extra for lattice
if you wish

Preheat oven to 375°F.

Steam parsnips until tender, about 20 minutes. Drain, cool enough to handle, and chop fine. Combine in a medium bowl with salt, honey, ginger, cinnamon, orange juice, orange rind (if used), and eggs. Mix well. Pour into pastry shell and top with lattice if desired. Bake 30 minutes.

Serves 8.

VEGETARIAN

PARSNIP PIE IS TRADITIONALLY MADE WITH A LATTICE CRUST AND DECORATED
WITH PRIMROSES, A CELEBRATION OF EARLY SPRING. IT IS A SIDE DISH RATHER
THAN A DESSERT AND GOES WELL WITH ROAST MEAT OR POULTRY.

potato watercress purée

2 bunches watercress, leaves only

2/3 cup whipping cream

2 pounds potatoes

salt and pepper

butter

1 tablespoon minced parsley

Put all but 1 tablespoon of watercress leaves in a colander. Immerse colander for 30 seconds in a large saucepan of boiling water. Transfer leaves to blender, add cream, and purée until smooth. Peel potatoes and boil until tender. Drain and mash, mixing in salt, pepper, and butter to taste. Add watercress cream and stir. Garnish with parsley and reserved watercress leaves.

Serves 4 to 6.

VEGETARIAN, GLUTEN-FREE

THE BRIGHT, BLANCHED WATERCRESS TURNS THESE MASHED POTATOES
INTO A REAL ST. PATRICK'S DAY GREEN. THE FLAVOR
IS FRESH RATHER THAN PEPPERY.

roast potatoes with rosemary

2 pounds potatoes, the smaller and younger the better, scrubbed and cut into 1-inch cubes

leaves from 4 large sprigs fresh rosemary

4 large cloves garlic, peeled and crushed

1/2 cup olive oil

salt and pepper

1 tablespoon chopped parsley

Preheat oven to 425°F.

Place potatoes, rosemary, and garlic in a roasting pan, pour olive oil over, and add salt and pepper to taste. Bake, stirring occasionally, until potatoes are browned and crisp on the outside, tender on the inside, about 30 to 40 minutes. Sprinkle with parsley and serve.

Serves 6.

VEGAN, GLUTEN-FREE

REALLY FRESH, NEW POTATOES ARE SWEET ENOUGH TO EAT RAW. YOU WON'T GET THAT KIND OF FLAVOR FROM WINTER STORAGE POTATOES, WHICH HAVE LONG SINCE CONVERTED THEIR SUGAR INTO STARCH, BUT THEY STILL CAN TASTE WONDERFUL WITHOUT A LOT OF FUSS OR SOUR CREAM. THIS DISH NEEDS FRESH HERBS. OREGANO (WHICH GROWS ALL WINTER IN MY GARDEN) CAN BE USED INSTEAD OF ROSEMARY. THE BEST POTATOES FOR ROASTING ARE THIN-SKINNED VARIETIES LIKE WHITE ROSE AND YELLOW FINN. BIG, FLOURY BAKING POTATOES WON'T WORK AS WELL.

colcannon

potatoes

cabbage

butter

salt & pepper

Boil separately some potatoes and cabbage. When done, drain and squeeze the cabbage, and chop, or mince it very small. Mash the potatoes, and mix them gradually but thoroughly with the chopped cabbage, adding butter, pepper and salt. There should be twice as much potato as cabbage.

VEGETARIAN, GLUTEN-FREE

An old Irish dish, with lots of variations. Similar recipes turn up in Wales, Scotland, England, and Holland. It shows up on a lot of Irish tables on Halloween and on Irish-American tables on St. Patrick's Day, along with the corned beef and soda bread. Our community chorus sings about it, too: "thinking of the days when troubles we knew not, and our mothers made colcannon in the little skillet pot." Precise measurements seem to violate the spirit of this kind of cooking, so herewith a recipe from a 19th-century American cookbook by Miss Eliza Leslie, quoted in James Beard's *American Cookery*. I would steam the cabbage instead of boiling it. Add some sausage, and you're on your way to another old Anglo Irish standby, Bubble and Squeak.

stampot

potatoes

kale, sauerkraut, or beets

butter

milk

salt & pepper

Add an equal portion of hot, mashed potatoes to hot, cooked kale, cabbage, sauerkraut, or chopped beets. Mash together, add some butter and a little milk, and salt and pepper to taste. This has made many a meal, perhaps with a little bacon or sausage on the side.

VEGETARIAN, GLUTEN-FREE

Stampot is to Dutch cooks what colcannon is to the Irish.

koftesi

2 pounds potatoes (about 6 medium), cooked and mashed

2 tablespoons melted butter

2 tablespoons chopped parsley

6 scallions or 3 slender leeks, white part only, chopped

1/2 cup canned plum tomatoes, drained, seeded, and chopped

1 cup fine dry bread crumbs

1/2 cup cottage cheese

1 egg, lightly beaten

salt and pepper

about 1/2 cup sifted flour

olive oil

Preheat oven to 400°F.

Coat a baking sheet with olive oil. Put mashed potatoes in a medium bowl and add, in order, butter, parsley, scallions, tomatoes, bread crumbs, cottage cheese, and egg, stirring after each addition. When mixture is well blended, add salt and pepper and work in just enough flour to make a stiff dough.

Press spoonfuls of dough into patties on a floured board, or pat into shape with your floured hands. Put patties on baking sheet, brush tops with olive oil, and bake until golden, about 15 minutes.

Makes 2 dozen 3-inch patties.

VEGETARIAN

THESE TURKISH POTATO PANCAKES ARE QUICK (IF YOU HAVE SOME LEFTOVER COOKED POTATOES), EASY, AND ATTRACTIVE, WITH CHEERFUL FLECKS OF RED AND GREEN. THEY MAKE A GOOD LUNCH ALONG WITH A BOWL OF SOUP OR A SALAD.

pumpkin-cheese pancakes

2 tablespoons butter or light oil

2 medium leeks or large scallions, sliced into rounds

2 cups grated peeled pumpkin or other winter squash

salt and pepper

1/4 teaspoon nutmeg

2 eggs

6 tablespoons milk

6 tablespoons flour

1/4 cup grated Jarlsberg or Parmesan cheese

Melt butter or oil in a heavy, medium-sized skillet over medium-low heat. Add leeks and stir 1 minute. Add pumpkin, salt, pepper, and nutmeg. Cook until pumpkin is tender, stirring frequently, about 5 minutes. Remove from heat and let cool while you start the batter.

Beat together eggs, milk, flour, and cheese. Add pumpkin mixture and blend. Butter a large, heavy skillet and heat to medium-high. Lower heat to medium and make small pancakes, using about 2 tablespoons of batter for each. Cook about 45 seconds per side. Serve on a warmed plate, sprinkled with a little more nutmeg.

*Serves 4 as a side dish or
2 as a main dish.*

VEGETARIAN

THESE LITTLE GOLDEN PANCAKES ARE A HIT AT OUR HOUSE WITH NO CONDIMENTS NECESSARY.
THEY COULD BE DRESSED UP WITH A SPOONFUL OF SOUR CREAM OR YOGURT.
I USE A BLENDER TO MIX THE INGREDIENTS. IF YOU ARE DOING IT BY HAND,
BE SURE TO COOK THE PUMPKIN UNTIL IT IS REALLY SOFT.

broiled radicchio

1/2 cup olive oil

2 cloves garlic, sliced

2 tablespoons fresh lemon juice

salt and pepper

2 medium heads radicchio

Preheat broiler to 450°F.

Heat olive oil in a small skillet, add garlic, and cook over low heat until garlic begins to turn color. Remove from heat and strain out garlic. Add lemon juice, salt, and pepper.

Cut radicchio in half lengthwise and brush surface with olive oil mixture. Place cut side down on a hot broiling pan. Cook 3 to 5 minutes, turning once, until radicchio is dull brown and edges are slightly crisped. Transfer to plates and pour remaining oil over the top.

Serves 4.

VEGAN, GLUTEN-FREE

THIS COULDN'T BE EASIER, AND IT MAKES AN EXCELLENT FOIL FOR THE MILD RISOTTOS
AND POLENTAS OF THE VENETO REGION OF ITALY, WHERE IT ORIGINATES.
IT'S ALSO A GOOD USE FOR SLIGHTLY RAGGED-LOOKING PLANTS.

le gourmand salsify

1 pound salsify or scorzonera

1 cup heavy cream

nutmeg

1/8 teaspoon white pepper

1 tablespoon chopped chervil, Italian parsley, or sweet cicely

salt

Peel salsify or scorzonera and cut into pieces the size of your little finger. Put cut pieces in acidulated water as you go. Drain, then steam until barely tender, about 5 minutes.

Combine cream, nutmeg, pepper, and herbs in a heavy, non-aluminum saucepan or sauté pan. Bring to a boil, lower heat, and cook gently until cream is reduced almost to the consistency of sauce. Add salsify or scorzonera and continue cooking until liquid makes a sauce. Add salt to taste.

Serves 3 or 4.

VEGETARIAN, GLUTEN-FREE

BRUCE NAFTALY AND ROBIN SAUNDERS SERVE THIS AS AN APPETIZER
AT LE GOURMAND IN SEATTLE.

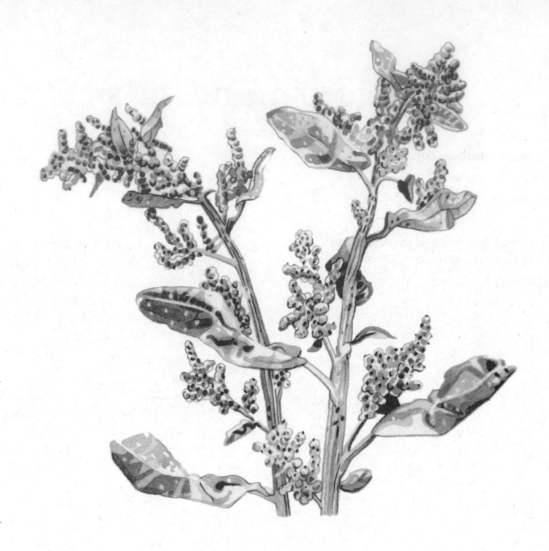

orache

· · · · · · · · · · · · · · · · · · ·

scorzonera with sour cream

2 pounds scorzonera (6 to 8 roots), peeled

1 medium onion, minced

2 tablespoons butter

1 tablespoon flour

1 cup sour cream or sour half-and-half

salt and pepper

2 tablespoons grated Swiss cheese

2 tablespoons bread crumbs

Preheat oven to 400°F.

Steam scorzonera until tender, about 8 minutes. Remove from heat and dice when cool enough to handle. Mix together scorzonera and onion and spoon into greased casserole. Melt butter in small saucepan. Stir in flour and simmer 1 minute. Add sour cream or sour half-and-half and salt and pepper to taste. Heat gently; don't let it boil. Spoon mixture over vegetables and toss lightly to blend. Sprinkle with grated Swiss cheese and crumbs. Bake 15 to 20 minutes.

Serves 4 to 6.

VEGETARIAN

THE FULL FLAVOR OF SCORZONERA (OR SALSIFY, ITS TASTE TWIN) CAN HOLD ITS OWN WITH THIS RICH SAUCE.

puréed sorrel

2 pounds (about 10 cups) of sorrel,
washed and stemmed

1/4 cup heavy cream

salt and pepper

nutmeg

⊱ cook's note

Don't use an aluminum or cast iron pan when cooking sorrel as it turns the greens a creepy blackish-brown.

Blanch sorrel for 2 to 3 minutes. Drain, press out excess water, and purée. Pour the purée into a deep saucepan, whisk in cream, and heat gently until mixture thickens. Season to taste with salt, pepper, and nutmeg.

Makes 2-1/2 cups.

VEGETARIAN, GLUTEN-FREE

SORREL COOKS SO QUICKLY THAT THIS USEFUL COMBINATION CAN BE READY IN MINUTES.
IT MAKES A GOOD SAUCE OR OMELET FILLING.

TWO POUNDS IS A WHOLE LOT OF SORREL, BUT NOT AN UNREASONABLE EXPECTATION
FOR AN ESTABLISHED GARDEN, AS THIS IS ONE OF HARDIEST OF PERENNIALS.
PROPORTIONS CAN BE CUT TO SUIT YOUR CROP.

shikumchee:
korean spinach and garlic

2 teaspoons sugar

3 tablespoons soy sauce

2 tablespoons toasted sesame seeds

1/4 cup minced scallions or small leeks

1 tablespoon toasted sesame seed oil

1 tablespoon minced garlic

2 pounds fresh spinach leaves

Combine all ingredients except spinach in a mixing bowl and blend well. Just before serving, steam spinach leaves over boiling water. Chop coarsely. Arrange on warm serving platter. Pour sauce over and serve immediately.

Serves 4.

VEGAN

DURING THE SEATTLE WORLD'S FAIR OF 1962, A FAMILY OF MUSICIANS OPENED WHAT I THINK WAS THE FIRST KOREAN RESTAURANT IN SEATTLE. I HAD THIS SPINACH THERE AS A CHILD, SERVED WITH ELEGANT METAL CHOPSTICKS, AND I NEVER FORGOT IT. ONCE THEY HAD PAID JULLIARD TUITION FOR THEIR CHILDREN, THE PARENTS CLOSED THE BUSINESS AND RETIRED. STEAMED CARROT MATCHSTICKS CAN BE TREATED THE SAME WAY, AND THEY LOOK NICE ON A PLATE WITH THE SPINACH.

dry spinach curry

1/4 cup ghee (*see page 236*) or mild oil

1 medium onion, chopped fine

2 cloves garlic, chopped fine

2 small green chilies, seeds and ribs removed, cut into 1/4-inch pieces

1 pound spinach, washed, drained, and coarsely chopped

salt and black pepper

Heat ghee or oil in heavy saucepan. Add onion and garlic and sauté until they begin to turn color, but do not let them brown. Add chilies and continue cooking a minute. Add spinach, turning constantly. Add a sprinkle of water if necessary. Add salt and pepper and cook until done.

Serves 3 or 4.

VEGAN, GLUTEN-FREE

THIS CURRY IS SERVED IN SMALL PORTIONS AS A CONDIMENT IN AN INDIAN MEAL.

spinach sesame purée

2 pounds spinach, washed and trimmed

2 tablespoons butter

2 tablespoons toasted sesame seeds

1 tablespoon chopped chives

Steam spinach until soft, drain thoroughly, chop, and purée. Melt butter in small saucepan over low heat. Stir in spinach and sesame seeds and cook until heated through. Remove from heat and blend in chives.

Serves 3 or 4.

VEGETARIAN, GLUTEN-FREE

THIS HAS THE FLAVOR OF JAPANESE SPINACH SALAD, WITH A MUCH DIFFERENT TEXTURE.

spinach with raisins and pine nuts

2 pounds spinach or chard

1/4 cup raisins

1/4 cup pine nuts

1/4 cup olive oil

2 garlic cloves, crushed and peeled

salt and pepper

Steam spinach or chard (about 5 minutes for spinach; 10 minutes for chard) and chop coarsely. Plump raisins in warm water and drain. Toss raisins and pine nuts with spinach or chard and set aside.

Heat oil in a large skillet and sauté garlic gently until cooked but not brown. Add greens, toss well, cover, and simmer for 5 minutes. Uncover and raise heat if necessary to evaporate excess moisture. Season to taste with salt and pepper and serve at once.

Serves 4.

VEGAN, GLUTEN-FREE

THIS COMBINATION, WHICH ALSO CAN BE MADE WITH CHARD, IS COMMON TO A NUMBER OF MEDITERRANEAN CUISINES. THE USE OF RAISINS WITH GREENS IS A SIGN OF NORTH AFRICAN INFLUENCE. A CATALONIAN VERSION ADDS 2 ANCHOVY FILLETS ALONG WITH THE GARLIC. COOK THEM GENTLY UNTIL THEY DISSOLVE. THE MILD RICHNESS OF THE PINE NUTS BINDS THE OTHER CONTRASTING FLAVORS TOGETHER AND MAKES THIS SIMPLE PREPARATION PERFECT.

polenta and sweet potatoes

1 cup polenta

3 cups water

1/2 teaspoon salt

2 medium yams or sweet potatoes

Bake sweet potatoes or yams, unpeeled, (I like garnet yams for the lovely color) at 400°F until very soft. Start checking after half an hour.

Meanwhile, boil the water in a heavy saucepan. Dribble in polenta, stirring constantly. Add salt. Reduce heat to simmer and cook for at least 1/2 hour, stirring every few minutes with a wooden spoon. Really work the spoon against the bottom of the pan so that the mixture doesn't adhere. When the polenta becomes a thick porridge (thicker than soup, thinner than mashed potatoes), add the yams. They should be soft enough to squeeze right out of their skins like toothpaste. Turn the heat to medium-low and cook another 2 or 3 minutes, stirring constantly.

Adjust salt to taste, stir in a tablespoon of good olive oil if you want, and serve. If you are adding cheese, do so while it's still hot.

Variation: Instead of yams, peel, slice, and then boil a medium celeriac until soft. Drain, reserving the water. Return the water to the saucepan, adding enough more water to equal 3 cups. Add the polenta and 1/2 teaspoon salt and cook as above. Purée the celeriac and add to polenta as above. Just before serving, stir in 1 tablespoon of good olive oil.

Serves 4.

VEGETARIAN, GLUTEN-FREE

A VERY SIMPLE SIDE DISH THAT CAN BE EITHER SWEET OR SAVORY. THE GENTLE SWEETNESS OF THE MIXTURE, WITH THE SLIGHT GRIT OF THE CORNMEAL, MADE ME THINK OF DESSERT PEARS AND CHEESE, SO I STIRRED IN ½ CUP OF GORGONZOLA. MY FRIEND ROBERT SAID IT WAS LIKE HIS WEST VIRGINIA CHILDHOOD GRITS, ONLY WAY BETTER, SO HE SKIPPED THE CHEESE AND POURED ON SOME MAPLE SYRUP.

sweet potatoes and apples with maple glaze

3 pounds baked sweet potatoes or yams

3 cooking apples

1/4 cup fresh lemon juice

4 tablespoons butter

1/4 cup firmly packed brown sugar

1/2 cup maple syrup

1/2 teaspoon cinnamon

2 tablespoons dark rum (optional)

Preheat oven to 400°F. Put rack at highest position.

Use some of the butter to prepare a large baking pan or gratin dish. Let sweet potatoes cool slightly, cut off ends, pull off peel with dull knife, and cut on the diagonal into 1/4-inch slices.

Peel and core apples and cut lengthwise into 1/2-inch slices. Put into a bowl and toss with lemon juice. Place in baking pan, overlapping slices slightly and making a nice pattern of sweet potato and apple.

Combine butter, sugar, maple syrup, cinnamon, and rum (if used) in a small saucepan and stir over medium heat until sugar dissolves. Pour mixture slowly over apples and sweet potatoes so that top is uniformly moistened. Bake in upper third of oven, basting frequently, for 25 minutes or until apples are tender and sweet potatoes have a nice glaze. Broil for 20 seconds if edges aren't browned.

Serves 6 to 8.

VEGETARIAN, GLUTEN-FREE

THE IDEA IS TO SET OFF THE SWEET POTATOES WITH A BIT OF APPLE TARTNESS
AND THEN BRING THE DISH TOGETHER WITH THE FLAVOR OF MAPLE SYRUP.
IT'S A GOOD PLAN, EASILY EXECUTED.

swiss chard and olives

2 pounds chard (stems removed), roughly chopped, or 1 pound each chard and spinach

4 tablespoons olive oil

2 cloves garlic, chopped

1 tablespoon sweet paprika

2 teaspoons turmeric

1/4 teaspoon pepper

6 large green or black Greek or Italian olives, pitted, rinsed, and chopped

rind of 1 preserved lemon (optional), rinsed and cut into thin wedges (*see page 217*)

Bring 1/2 cup water to a boil in a saucepan, add chard, reduce heat, and simmer, covered, until tender, about 10 minutes. Drain. If you are using both chard and spinach, cook the spinach separately for about 5 minutes in the water that remains on the leaves after washing. Drain well.

Heat oil in a heavy saucepan or skillet. Add garlic and sauté over medium heat for 1 minute. Add paprika, turmeric, and pepper and mix well. Add greens and olives and toss to blend thoroughly. Continue cooking, stirring constantly, for 3 or 4 minutes. Add preserved lemon (if used), cook another 2 minutes, and serve hot.

VEGAN, GLUTEN-FREE

THE EMPHATIC FLAVORS OF PROVENÇAL AND NORTH AFRICAN CUISINES GO WELL WITH TOUGH WINTER CHARD. THE TIANS OF PROVENCE COMBINE CHARD WITH ANCHOVIES OR EVEN SALT COD. MOROCCAN DISHES, SUCH AS THIS ONE, USE PUNGENT OLIVES AND PRESERVED LEMONS. WIDELY USED IN NORTH AFRICA, PRESERVED LEMONS WERE AT ONE TIME A CRAZE IN THE US. (DOES ANYONE REMEMBER WHEN AMY'S LOVE OF PICKLED LEMONS GOT HER INTO TROUBLE IN *LITTLE WOMEN*?) THEY ARE QUICK TO PREPARE, BUT THEY SHOULD CURE FOR A MONTH BEFORE USING. THIS RECIPE IS GOOD—THOUGH NOT THE SAME—WITHOUT THEM. DO NOT SUBSTITUTE FRESH LEMON.

preserved lemons

5 or 6 small, thin-skinned organic lemons or limes

1/3 cup salt

juice of 2 lemons

Cut lemons or limes almost through from the blossom end into quarters, leaving them in one piece at the stem end. Sprinkle each with 1 teaspoon of salt and fit it together again. Place fruit in a sterilized 1-quart wide-mouth glass jar, squeezing snugly to fit. Add remaining salt, lemon juice, and enough warm water to cover. Close jar and shake to dissolve salt. Let stand for a month in a dark place. Don't worry if the lemons get a bit scummy; the scum is harmless, and it rinses off. These will keep for up to a year. You can use just the skin, as is traditional, or the whole lemon.

Serves 4.

VEGAN, GLUTEN-FREE

moroccan squash purée

2 tablespoons olive oil

1-1/2 pounds winter squash, peeled, seeded, and cut into 1-inch cubes

3 cloves garlic, chopped

1/2 cup water

1 tablespoon chopped parsley

1 tablespoon chopped cilantro

pinch of saffron (optional), crumbled in 1/4 cup warm water

1 teaspoon ground ginger

1/4 cup lemon juice

1 tablespoon sugar

1/4 teaspoon cayenne

salt and pepper

1 tablespoon ground cumin

Heat olive oil in a wide saucepan or skillet. Add squash, garlic, and water. Cover and cook, stirring frequently, for 15 to 20 minutes or until squash is tender. Combine rest of ingredients except cumin. Pour over squash and simmer, covered, another 10 minutes. Add a little water if necessary to prevent sticking. The squash will start to disintegrate.

Sprinkle with cumin and serve warm.

Serves 4.

VEGAN, GLUTEN-FREE

WHEN I FIRST STARTED BRINGING THIS TO POTLUCKS, MORE THAN 20 YEARS AGO, PEOPLE HAD ALL KINDS OF TROUBLE GUESSING THE MAIN INGREDIENT THAT MELDED SO BEAUTIFULLY WITH THE HERBS AND SPICES. (THEY DIDN'T SEEM TO MIND GOING BACK FOR MORE WHILE THEY TRIED TO FIGURE IT OUT.) NOW THE IDEA OF A SAVORY WINTER SQUASH DISH IS MORE FAMILIAR, AND NONE THE WORSE FOR THAT. IT'S A GREAT DISH FOR A COLD DAY.

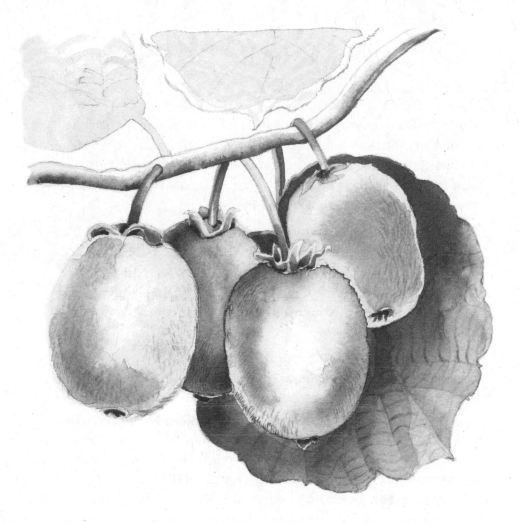

kiwi

· · · · · · · · · · ·

kiwi description, p. 21

RISOTTOS

My taste for risotto was established while studying in Italy as an already food-obsessed 19-year-old. My understanding of its basic structure came much later, from the wonderful and non-intimidating book *Risotto*, by Judith Barrett and Norma Wasserman, which I highly recommend.

Risottos are a particular boon to winter gardeners because they can transform a weather-beaten selection of heterogeneous vegetables into a civilized and delicious dish. As long as you have a well-made sofritto, a flavorful stock, and the right variety of rice, almost all other ingredients, from squid ink to grapefruit, are negotiable.

The sofritto is the base flavoring, consisting of fat—generally butter or olive oil—and onions, plus whatever other finely minced ingredients will fit the particular variety. The stock can be poultry, meat, fish, or vegetable, once again depending on the dish. The rice must be short grain and glutinous but not all the way to sticky. Arborio rice, originally grown in the Po Valley of northern Italy, is the standard. If you use "regular" long-grain rice you may have a tasty side dish, but it won't be risotto. The seductive creamy richness, which combines so enticingly with the al dente texture of each rice grain, comes from the combination of rice variety and cooking technique. It is the main reason that a risotto, although actually low in fat, still tastes rich and luscious.

carrot and radicchio risotto

5 cups vegetable or chicken stock

1/2 cup dry white wine

3 tablespoons olive oil or a combination of olive oil and butter

1/3 cup finely chopped onion

1-1/2 cups arborio rice

1 cup finely chopped radicchio

1 cup matchstick cut carrots

1 tablespoon chopped parsley

1/2 cup grated Parmesan cheese

Bring broth to a simmer in a medium saucepan.

While broth is heating, warm the oil or oil and butter mixture in a heavy saucepan over moderate heat. Add the onion and sauté for 1 or 2 minutes. Do not let it brown. Add rice to the sofritto mixture and stir until the rice is coated with the sofritto. Add the wine and stir until it is absorbed.

Stir in the radicchio and carrots and add the broth, 1/2 cup at a time, stirring after each addition until liquid is absorbed. Total cooking time is about 20 minutes. When the rice is al dente, add the last 1/4 cup of broth and the remaining ingredients. Stir in well and serve warm.

Serves 4.

THE SWEETNESS OF CARROTS AND THE SLIGHT BITE OF RADICCHIO, ORANGE AND PINKISH
FLECKS IN THE CREAMY RICE, WITH JUST A BIT OF RESISTANCE. IT'S VEGETABLE ALCHEMY.
GOOD BROTH IS IMPORTANT. THIS IS A FINE TIME TO USE HOMEMADE STOCK,
IN WHICH CASE THE RISOTTO IS RELIABLY GLUTEN-FREE.

chestnut risotto

1 pound fresh chestnuts or
1/2 pound dried

1 bay leaf

2 medium leeks, white part only, or
1 small onion, minced

4 tablespoons butter, divided

1-1/2 cups arborio rice

3 cups beef or vegetable stock

1/2 cup half and half

3 tablespoons grated Parmesan cheese

Soak dried chestnuts for 1 hour in lukewarm water. Skip the soaking if you have fresh nuts. Cut an X on the flat of each shell and simmer with bay leaf for 20 to 30 minutes. Cool, peel, and crumble into a small bowl.

Bring broth to a simmer in a medium saucepan. While the stock is heating, melt 2 tablespoons of the butter in a medium saucepan and sauté leeks or onion until translucent. Add rice and half of the crumbled chestnuts and sauté about 2 minutes.

Pour in stock 1/2 cup at a time, stirring, until each addition is absorbed. Meanwhile, heat half-and-half in a small pan. Add the remaining chestnuts and cook over very low heat for 5 minutes. Mash a few of the chestnuts in the half-and-half, stir, and add mixture to rice along with the Parmesan cheese and the remaining 2 tablespoons of butter. Serve warm.

Serves 4.

INTRIGUING AND DELICIOUS, THIS CONTEMPORARY ITALIAN DISH GOES WELL
WITH CHICKEN, BUT WE LIKE IT AS A MAIN DISH.

rutabaga mashed potatoes

2 medium rutabagas (4 to 6 inches long)

2 medium baking potatoes (there should be about equal quantities of rutabagas and potatoes)

2 cloves garlic, minced

1 small to medium onion, diced

4 tablespoons olive oil

3 tablespoons Worcestershire sauce

salt, pepper, and butter to taste

1/2 cup grated goat cheese (I like the goat Gouda from Gothberg Farms, just a few miles south.)

Peel and cube the potatoes. Cut off the ends of the rutabagas, cut into 1/2-thick slices, and peel off the outer rind. Cube to match the potatoes. Steam vegetables until soft. Do not overcook.

Meanwhile, heat the olive oil in a skillet or heavy saucepan, add garlic and onion, and cook slowly until soft and golden. Depending on the moisture content of the onion, this could take as much as 30 minutes. Add Worcestershire sauce, combine the onion/garlic mixture with the vegetables, and mash.

Stir in salt, pepper, and butter to taste. Pass the grated cheese.

Bill says this goes especially well with a burgundy or other heavy red wine, and I believe him.

Serves 4.

VEGETARIAN (DEPENDING ON THE WORCESTERSHIRE SAUCE)

FOR A RUNDOWN ON CLASSIC DELICIOUS WAYS TO USE ROOT VEGETABLES AS ACCOMPANIMENTS TO EQUALLY CLASSIC SERVINGS OF RED MEAT, YOU CAN'T DO BETTER THAN *MASTERING THE ART OF FRENCH COOKING*. IT WON'T COME AS A SURPRISE THAT THE COMMON DENOMINATOR IN ALL THOSE RECIPES IS A WHOLE LOT OF BUTTER. I HAVEN'T INCLUDED MANY DISHES OF THIS STYLE, SINCE MY IDEA IS GENERALLY TO PUT WINTER VEGETABLES IN STARRING RATHER THAN SUPPORTING ROLES. HOWEVER, THIS IS ONE VERSION THAT I COULDN'T RESIST. I GOT IT FROM MY PEN PAL BILL BOWES, WHO LEARNED IT FROM SOMEONE FROM VERMONT, "WHERE THEY KNOW ROOTS."

oven-roasted sweet potatoes

6 tablespoons butter

1 clove garlic, sliced

two 8-ounce yams or 2 medium sweet potatoes

4 tablespoons soy sauce

2 tablespoons balsamic vinegar

2 tablespoons sugar

dash of hot pepper sauce

Melt butter in a small saucepan. Add garlic and remove from heat. Let stand 15 minutes.

Preheat oven to 375°F.

Peel yams and cut lengthwise into wedges. Remove garlic from butter and discard. Pour butter into baking dish. Add yams, turning to coat evenly with butter. Bake 30 minutes.

Meanwhile, combine soy sauce, balsamic vinegar, sugar, and hot pepper sauce in a small bowl. Stir until sugar is dissolved. Brush over yams and bake another 15 to 20 minutes until tender.

Serves 4.

VEGETARIAN

I USUALLY MIX MY SWEET POTATOES WITH OTHER VEGETABLES BEFORE ROASTING,
BUT ONCE IN A WHILE IT'S NICE TO CONCENTRATE ON ONE VEGETABLE FLAVOR AT A TIME.
THE VINEGAR/SOY/HOT PEPPER COMBO ELIMINATES ANY DANGER OF CLOYING SWEETNESS.
THIS IS RICHER THAN MOST ROASTED VEGGIE TREATMENTS, BUT YOU COULD REDUCE
OR EVEN SKIP THE BUTTER AND STILL HAVE AN EXCELLENT DISH.

baked sweet potato snack strips

sweet potatoes

olive oil

spice mix or dry seasoning

Preheat oven to 400°F.

Cut raw sweet potato into julienne strips. Pour a little olive oil into your palm and rub onto the sweet potatoes. Sprinkle with your favorite dry seasoning—I favor Cajun spice—and mix that in too. Spread sweet potatoes in a single layer on bakers parchment or a silicon mat. Bake until some of the pieces start to brown. Serve hot.

VEGAN, GLUTEN-FREE

THESE ARE NOT THE HOME EQUIVALENT OF SWEET POTATO FRIES, BUT THEY ARE
LOWER IN FAT, VERY VERY EASY, AND THEY GO JUST AS FAST.

swiss chard parmigiana

12 to 16 large chard stalks (from about 2 pounds of fresh chard), blanched and cut into 4-inch lengths

salt and pepper

1/2 to 2/3 cup grated Parmesan cheese

6 tablespoons melted butter

Preheat oven to 400°F. Butter a 9-by-12-inch baking dish and make a single layer of drained chard stems. Season with salt and pepper and sprinkle with 1/3 of the cheese and a drizzle of butter. Make two more layers in this manner, saving enough cheese and butter for a good coating on top. Bake 20 minutes or until top is golden. Let stand 10 minutes or so before serving.

Serves 4.

VEGETARIAN, GLUTEN-FREE

MOST CHARD RECIPES CALL FOR THE LEAVES ONLY, BUT SOME CUISINES VALUE
THE WIDE STEMS ENOUGH TO RAISE SPECIAL BROAD-STEMMED VARIETIES.
BLANCHING REMOVES THE SOMEWHAT METALLIC FLAVOR OF OLDER SPECIMENS.

swiss chard stalks beurre noir

12 to 16 large chard stalks, cut into 4-inch lengths

3 tablespoons butter

1/2 teaspoon finely chopped fresh sage

pepper

1/2 teaspoon lemon juice

Steam chard stalks until barely tender. Heat butter in a medium skillet, stirring constantly until it starts to brown. Add sage, pepper, and lemon juice and pour over chard stalks.

Serves 4.

VEGETARIAN, GLUTEN-FREE

IF YOU HAVE FRESH SAGE, SAUTÉ IT UNTIL IT STARTS TO GET CRISP. THE SALT IN THE BUTTER MAY BE ENOUGH FOR THE DISH. IF NOT, SALT TO TASTE.

turnips with anchovies

3 tablespoons olive oil

4 garlic cloves, sliced thin

3 anchovy fillets, drained and cut into small pieces

2 tablespoons fresh rosemary or 1 tablespoon dried

2 pounds turnips, peeled and sliced thin

salt and pepper to taste

1 tablespoon minced parsley

Heat oil in saucepan or medium skillet. Add garlic, anchovies, and rosemary and sauté over medium-low heat for 1 minute. Don't let the garlic brown.

Add turnips, season with salt and pepper, and sauté, stirring frequently, until tender, about 8 to 10 minutes. Sprinkle with parsley and serve hot.

Serves 6.

THIS ITALIAN DISH IS BEST WITH SMALL YOUNG TURNIPS, BUT IT WORKS FINE WITH BIGGER ONES PROVIDED THEIR FLAVOR IS GOOD. OLD, HOT, CORKY TURNIPS ARE NO GOOD FOR THIS (OR ANYTHING ELSE). THE SAME RECIPE, MINUS THE ROSEMARY, CAN BE USED FOR TURNIP GREENS.

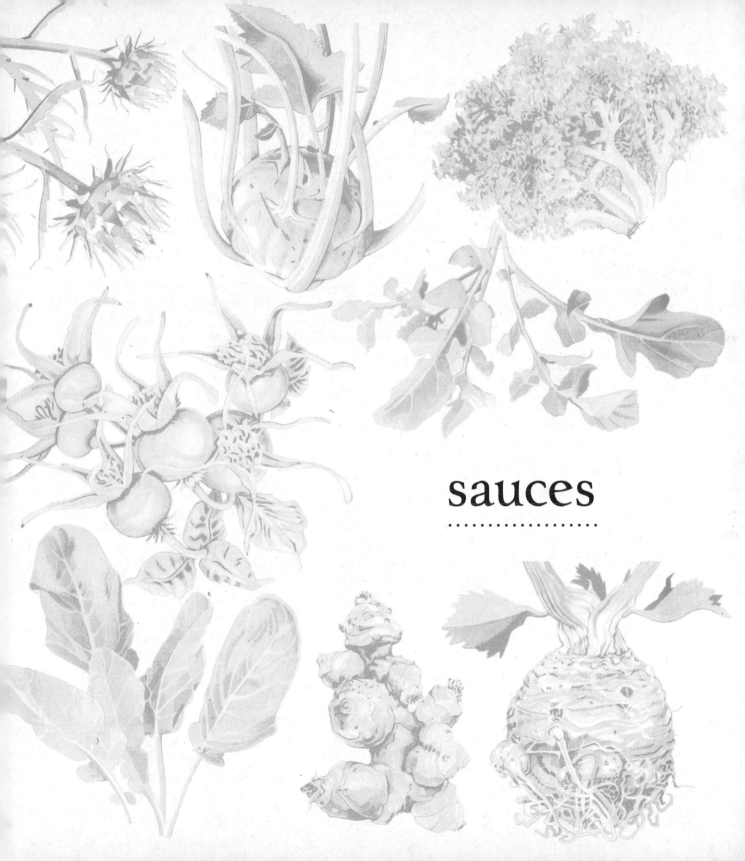

sauces

skordalia

1 pound russet or other baking potatoes

yolk of one large egg

1/2 cup olive oil

4–5 garlic cloves

juice of 2 lemons

1/2 teaspoon salt

Scrub the unpeeled potatoes. Put them in a saucepan with water to cover, bring to a boil, and then reduce heat and cook, covered, until soft. Drain and cool enough to peel. Put the peeled potatoes in a medium bowl and mash with a fork or potato masher.

Pound garlic to a paste in a mortar or pulse with a food processor. Add egg yolk, garlic, olive oil, lemon juice, and salt to the mashed potatoes and stir until well blended. Thin with some fish or vegetable stock if desired.

Makes 2 cups.

VEGETARIAN, GLUTEN-FREE

THIS PUNGENT GREEK SAUCE IS SOMEWHERE BETWEEN MASHED POTATOES AND MAYONNAISE. I'VE TRIED A NUMBER OF VERSIONS, AND THIS IS MY FAVORITE. HOWEVER, THE EGG YOLK IS OPTIONAL, SO A VEGAN VERSION IS JUST FINE. FOR A POURABLE SAUCE, YOU CAN KEEP GOING WITH THE OLIVE OIL OR ADD SOME STOCK; FISH STOCK IS RECOMMENDED, BUT ONCE AGAIN, VEGETABLE STOCK WILL BE GOOD TOO. ANOTHER COMMON ADDITION IS ⅓ TO ½ CUP GROUND NUTS. WALNUTS, ALMONDS OR PINE NUTS ALL SHOW UP IN DIFFERENT RECIPES. STILL OTHER RECIPES INCLUDE BREAD CRUMBS, BUT I HAVEN'T LIKED THOSE AS MUCH. AS LONG AS YOU HAVE POTATOES, OLIVE OIL, GARLIC, AND LEMON JUICE, YOU ARE TRUE TO THE IDEA OF SKORDALIA

I MAKE IT BY POUNDING THE GARLIC IN A MORTAR AND MASHING THE POTATOES WITH A FORK. YOU CAN ALSO USE AN EGGBEATER OR BLENDER, BUT THE SAME CAUTIONS APPLY AS WITH OTHER MASHED POTATO DISHES. GRAINY (NOT LUMPY) IS GOOD, GLUEY IS NOT, SO DON'T OVER PROCESS. DO NOT USE FINGERLINGS, YUKON GOLDS, OR OTHER BOILING POTATOES HERE.

asian pear and jerusalem artichoke chutney

4 medium Asian pears, cored and sliced thin (2–3 cups)

1 cup sliced Jerusalem artichokes (I prefer the flavor of the red fuseaus)

3 scallions or small leeks, sliced thin

3 tablespoons lime juice

1 tablespoon rice vinegar

1/4 cup cilantro leaves

dash of hot sauce to taste

Combine the first 5 ingredients, getting the vinegar and lime juice on the fruits and veggies right away so they don't discolor. Add the cilantro and hot sauce and mix in gently.

Serves 4 to 6 depending on its role in the meal.

VEGAN, GLUTEN-FREE

I'M NOT ACTUALLY SURE WHAT TO CALL THIS: A CHUTNEY? A SALAD? A SALSA? MY SON-IN-LAW SAYS HE'S GOING TO PURÉE IT AS A MARINADE FOR PORK CHOPS, SO THERE'S ANOTHER OPTION. OBVIOUSLY IT'S VERSATILE, AND IT'S ALSO DELICIOUS, ESPECIALLY IN WINTER WHEN THESE BRIGHT FLAVORS ARE LESS COMMON.

wild sorrel
and nettle sauce

3 tablespoons minced shallots

3 tablespoons unsalted butter

1 large clove garlic, minced

24 wild sorrel leaves, or 15 leaves of cultivated sorrel

24 young nettle leaves

2 cups fish stock

1/4 cup dry white wine

1 cup heavy cream

3 tablespoons cold unsalted butter, in small pieces

Melt butter in a saucepan and sauté shallots and garlic until soft. Add sorrel and nettles and sauté gently for about a minute. Add fish stock and wine and bring to a boil. Boil gently until liquid is reduced by half. Purée mixture in blender and then pass through a fine sieve. Pour back into pot and add cream. Simmer 5 minutes or until thickened. Remove from heat and whisk in cold butter.

Spoon sauce onto plates and arrange seafood on top.

Makes 2 cups.

THE CHEFS AT SOOKE HARBOUR HOUSE SERVE THIS SAUCE WITH SAUTÉED ABALONE.
TRY IT ALSO WITH SCALLOPS, SHRIMP OR FISH.

niter kibbeh: clarified butter with spices

1 pound unsalted butter

4 tablespoons chopped onion

1-1/2 tablespoons chopped garlic

2 teaspoons grated fresh ginger

1/2 teaspoon turmeric

2 whole cardamom seeds, crushed, or 1/2 teaspoon ground cardamom

1-inch stick of cinnamon

2 or 3 whole cloves

1/8 teaspoon ground nutmeg

Slowly melt butter in a saucepan and then bring it to a boil. When butter is covered with foam, add all remaining ingredients, lower heat, and simmer, uncovered, over very low heat until the surface is transparent and the milk solids are on the bottom. This can take up to an hour. Pour off the clear liquid (leaving as much residue as possible in the pan) and strain through a double layer of damp cheesecloth. Strain twice more if you expect to keep the niter kibbeh for more than a few weeks. After three strainings, it should keep for two to three months, even at room temperature.

Makes about 2 cups.

VEGETARIAN, GLUTEN-FREE

LIKE INDIAN GHEE, THIS ETHIOPIAN PREPARATION SOLVES THE PROBLEM OF STORING BUTTER WITHOUT REFRIGERATION. YOU PROBABLY DON'T HAVE TO WORRY ABOUT THAT, BUT IF YOU WANT TO TURN THE SIMPLEST STEAMED VEGETABLES OR BOILED POTATOES INTO SOMETHING SPECIAL, LOOK NO FURTHER.

cranberry horseradish relish

1/2 pound cranberries

1/2 cup light brown sugar

1/4 cup grated fresh or bottled horseradish

2 tablespoons fresh lemon juice

Chop cranberries medium fine. (The job will be easier if you freeze them first.) Stir in remaining ingredients and mix well. Refrigerate for at least 2 days before serving.

Makes 2 cups.

VEGAN

TWO CUPS IS A LOT OF RELISH, BUT THIS TANGY COMBINATION IMPROVES WITH AGE. IT IS A RUSSIAN RECIPE, MEANT FOR BOILED BEEF OR POT ROAST. IT'S ALSO SENSATIONAL ON A BROILED SWISS CHEESE SANDWICH. USE FRESH HORSERADISH IF YOU POSSIBLY CAN.

pickled jerusalem artichokes

2 cups sliced Jerusalem artichokes

your favorite vinegar

Peel Jerusalem artichokes and slice thin. Keep peeled artichokes in acidulated water and return slices to acidulated water. When finished, drain and place slices in a glass jar. Pour vinegar over to cover. Refrigerate, covered, for at least 5 days before using. The pickles will keep indefinitely.

Makes 2 cups.

VEGAN, GLUTEN-FREE

A SIMPLE CONDIMENT, GOOD IN SALADS, FROM BRUCE NAFTALY AT LE GOURMAND IN SEATTLE. NAFTALY USES AN AGED SHERRY VINEGAR. YOU MIGHT WANT TO MAKE A FEW TEST BATCHES BEFORE SETTLING ON THE RIGHT FLAVOR FOR YOUR KITCHEN.

broccoli sauce

2 cups cooked broccoli

1/3 cup olive oil

1/3 cup red vinegar or balsamic vinegar

1/2 teaspoon basil

1/4 teaspoon cumin

salt and pepper

1 tablespoon tomato sauce

Combine all ingredients and purée. Reheat gently in small saucepan if broccoli is cold.

Serves 4.

VEGAN

THIS IS A GOOD USE FOR LEFTOVER BROCCOLI OR FOR THOSE LAST SIDE SHOOTS IN THE GARDEN THAT ARE TOO SKINNY TO SERVE ON THEIR OWN. SERVE OVER BROWN RICE OR A SUBSTANTIAL PASTA. FOLLOW WITH A CUSTARD OR A CLAFOUTI FOR A SIMPLE, HIGH-PROTEIN VEGETARIAN MEAL.

gremolata

1/2 cup minced Italian parsley

1 or 2 cloves minced garlic

1-1/2 teaspoons lemon zest

1/4 cup fine bread crumbs

salt and pepper to taste

Combine ingredients in a heavy bowl and mash with a mortar or the back of a spoon.

Makes 3/4 cup.

VEGAN.

GREMOLATA IS AN ITALIAN CONDIMENT DESIGNED TO BRIGHTEN UP FRIED FOODS. IT IS ALSO EXCELLENT WITH GRILLED MEATS AND FISH. MORE DELICATE FLAVORS CAN BE EASILY OVERWHELMED BY THE RAW GARLIC, SO YOU MAY WANT TO ADJUST PROPORTIONS ACCORDINGLY. THIS IS A STRIPPED DOWN VERSION, WHICH CAN BE AUGMENTED TO YOUR TASTE.

mint chutney

1/2 cup fresh mint leaves

1/2 cup cilantro

handful of roasted peanuts or cashews

3 or 4 cloves garlic

juice of 2 limes

2 teaspoons coriander seeds, crushed

1 tablespoon sugar

1 mildly hot pepper

pinch of cayenne

Combine all ingredients in blender or food processor and whirl until well mixed. Pour into a clean jar and cover tightly.

Makes about 1 cup.

VEGETARIAN

A REFRESHING EAST AFRICAN SAUCE FOR GRILLED FISH AND CHICKEN OR SEAFOOD CURRIES (AND IT'S ALSO GOOD WITH MARINATED TOFU). IT WILL KEEP SEVERAL WEEKS REFRIGERATED IN A TIGHTLY CLOSED JAR.

garam masala

cinnamon sticks

cardamom pods

cloves

The three basic ingredients of garam masala are cinnamon sticks, cardamom pods, and cloves in equal weights. Spread them on a baking sheet or pie plate and bake about 30 minutes at 200°F. Don't let them scorch. Remove from the oven, shell the cardamom and discard the pods, break the cinnamon sticks, and pulverize the spices in a blender or a coffee grinder (unless you want true village authenticity, in which case you will grind them by hand with a mortar and pestle). Other common additions are mace, coriander seeds, cumin, and black pepper. Dry garam masala keeps for months at room temperature provided the container is tightly closed.

VEGAN, GLUTEN-FREE

REFERRING TO INDIAN GARAM MASALAS IS A BIT LIKE TALKING ABOUT SALSAS OR MOLES IN MEXICAN COOKING. THERE ARE SO MANY VERSIONS THAT A SINGLE TERM CANNOT SUM THEM UP. UBIQUITOUS IN SOUTH ASIAN COOKING, MASALAS ARE VARIED TO SUIT THE DISH—SOMETIMES A POWDER, SOMETIMES A PASTE. YOU CAN FIND IT IN INDIAN STORES AND SPECIALTY GROCERIES. IT IS NOT AS LIKELY AS CURRY POWDER TO OVERWHELM A SIMPLE VEGETABLE CURRY. IF YOU SUBSTITUTE CURRY POWDER IN RECIPES THAT CALL FOR GARAM MASALA, YOU MIGHT WANT TO CUT BACK ON ANY ADDITIONAL CUMIN, TURMERIC OR CHILI POWDER.

ghee: clarified butter

unsalted butter

cheesecloth

Melt at least one stick of unsalted butter in a shallow pot over very low heat. It must not brown. Use a diffuser if you have an overeager gas range. Skim the froth that rises to the top, repeating the process until you have a clear, yellowish liquid. Cool a few minutes, pour off the clear liquid, and strain through at least 4 layers of cheesecloth to catch the last solid particles. Refrigerate in a covered jar. The ghee will solidify. Warm gently to liquefy before using it as oil.

GHEE IS THE COOKING OIL OF CHOICE IN MANY INDIAN RECIPES. IT IS SIMPLY BUTTER THAT HAS GONE THROUGH AN ADDITIONAL ROUND OF MELTING AND CLARIFYING TO REMOVE THE LAST BITS OF MILK SOLIDS. THE SOLIDS ARE WHAT CAUSE BUTTER TO SMOKE AT RELATIVELY LOW COOKING TEMPERATURES AND EVENTUALLY TO GO RANCID. THEY ALSO ARE THE ELEMENT THAT CAUSES TROUBLE FOR PEOPLE WHO ARE LACTOSE INTOLERANT. THE AMOUNT OF MILK SOLIDS LEFT IN COMMERCIAL BUTTER VARIES, AND MANY PEOPLE WHO CANNOT TOLERATE MILK BY THE GLASS CAN USE REGULAR BUTTER, BUT FOR THOSE WHO ARE MORE SENSITIVE STILL, GHEE COULD BE AN ANSWER. GHEE IS MORE WIDELY AVAILABLE COMMERCIALLY THAN IT WAS WHEN I WROTE THE FIRST *WINTER HARVEST*, BUT RURAL RESIDENTS MAY STILL HAVE TROUBLE BUYING IT, AND IT IS MUCH CHEAPER TO MAKE YOUR OWN. THOUGH SIMPLE, IT IS A BIT TIME CONSUMING, SO YOU MIGHT AS WELL WORK WITH AT LEAST A POUND OF BUTTER AT A TIME. IT KEEPS INDEFINITELY.

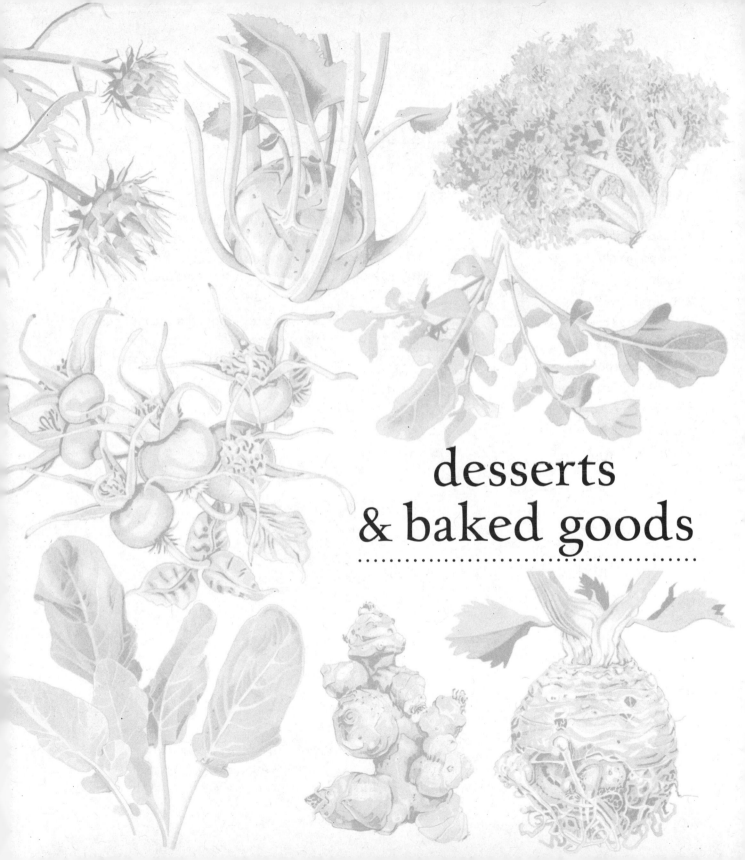

desserts
& baked goods

celeriac bread

3 cups flour

1/4 teaspoon baking powder

1 teaspoon baking soda

1 teaspoon salt

3 eggs

2/3 cup oil

2 cups grated celeriac

1/2 cup minced onion

1 tablespoon parsley

1/4 teaspoon dried marjoram

1/8 teaspoon pepper

butter

1 tablespoon flour

Preheat oven to 350°F.

Sift together flour, baking powder, baking soda, and salt. In large bowl, beat eggs and then add oil, celeriac, onion, parsley, marjoram, and pepper, beating until well blended. Add flour mixture a little at a time, mixing thoroughly after each addition.

Butter and flour two loaf pans. Spoon batter into pans, smooth tops, and bake 40 minutes or until a tester comes out clean. Cool 10 minutes and remove from pan.

Makes 2 loaves.

VEGETARIAN

I BROUGHT THIS SAVORY BREAD TO A POTLUCK AND WATCHED PEOPLE GO BACK
FOR SLICE AFTER SLICE AS THEY TRIED TO FIGURE OUT THE SECRET INGREDIENTS.
THE TEXTURE IS LIGHT AND FLAKY, RATHER LIKE THAT OF A BISCUIT.

squash muffins

2 cups flour

2 teaspoons baking powder

1 teaspoon baking soda

1/2 teaspoon salt

1 teaspoon cinnamon

1/2 teaspoon ground ginger

2 eggs

1/2 cup yogurt

1/4 cup light oil

3/4 cup light brown sugar

1 cup fresh squash or pumpkin purée

1/2 cup coarsely chopped dates

cook's note

The purée for this recipe should be relatively dry. If yours is more like applesauce, heat it gently in a wide saucepan or skillet, stirring frequently, until it wants to stick to the bottom.

Preheat oven to 450°F.

Combine flour, baking powder, baking soda, salt, cinnamon, and ginger in a large bowl. Beat eggs and yogurt together in a separate bowl; beat in oil and brown sugar. Stir in squash or pumpkin purée and mix thoroughly. Add to dry ingredients and mix well. Stir in dates. Pour into well-greased muffin tins and bake 20 to 25 minutes.

Makes 12 muffins.

VEGETARIAN

SQUASH PURÉE AND CHOPPED DATES GIVE THESE MUFFINS A RICH,
SWEET TASTE, GREAT FOR BREAKFAST.

quick herbed biscuits

1-1/4 cup all-purpose white flour

1/2 cup whole wheat flour

3 teaspoons baking powder

1/2 teaspoon salt

4 tablespoons butter or shortening, chilled

1 cup milk

1/4 cup watercress leaves, chopped very fine

1 tablespoon chopped parsley

1 tablespoon chopped chives

Preheat oven to 450°F.

Sift flours, baking powder and salt into a bowl. Cut in butter or shortening until mixture resembles coarse cornmeal. Make a well in the center and pour in milk. Stir briefly, and then stir in watercress, parsley, and chives. Drop dough by spoonfuls onto a greased baking sheet. Bake 10 to 12 minutes or until lightly browned.

Makes 18 small biscuits.

VEGETARIAN

WHEN IT COMES TO BISCUITS, I AM VERY WILLING TO SACRIFICE UNIFORMITY FOR SPEED. THESE LITTLE GEMS REQUIRE NO KNEADING OR ROLLING AND ARE NONE THE WORSE FOR LOOKING ROUGH-CUT. IF YOU PREFER ROLLED BISCUITS, DECREASE THE MILK TO ¾ CUP AND PROCEED AS USUAL.

carrot date squares

6 tablespoons melted butter

1 cup flour

1 cup sugar

1/2 teaspoon baking soda

1/4 teaspoon salt

1 teaspoon ground cinnamon

1/4 teaspoon freshly grated nutmeg

1/4 teaspoon ground ginger

1 large egg, beaten

1/2 cup plain yogurt

1/2 teaspoon vanilla

1 cup shredded carrots

1/2 cup coarsely chopped dates

Preheat oven to 375°F.

Grease an 11-by-14-inch baking dish. In large mixing bowl, combine flour, sugar, baking soda, and salt. Add cinnamon, nutmeg, and ginger and blend thoroughly. Gradually stir in melted butter. Add egg, yogurt, and vanilla. Blend well.

Stir in carrots and dates and pour into prepared pan. Bake 25 to 30 minutes or until a tester comes out clean. Cool briefly on rack and serve warm or cool.

Makes one large pan.

VEGETARIAN

THESE ARE SENSATIONAL. MAKE THEM IN A SMALLER PAN IF YOU WANT A CAKIER TEXTURE.

fruit pizza

DOUGH

5 tablespoons milk

1 teaspoon yeast

2-1/2 cups unbleached all-purpose flour

1 large egg

1/2 cup sugar

1/4 cup softened butter

TOPPING

1/2 cup raisins

1/2 cup fresh orange juice, divided

4 tablespoons Cointreau or Grand Marnier, divided

3 ripe Comice or Anjou pears

1/3 cup pine nuts

Dough

Scald milk and cool to tepid. Add yeast and set aside for 10 minutes. When yeast mixture is bubbling, combine with flour, egg, sugar, and butter. Turn onto a lightly floured board and knead about 5 minutes. Put dough in a large bowl, cover, and let rise in a warm, draft-free place until double, about 2 hours.

Topping

Put raisins in small mixing bowl. Add 3 tablespoons of the orange juice and 1 tablespoon of the Cointreau or Grand Marnier and set aside. Peel and core pears and cut into wedges 1/4-inch thick. Mix gently with remaining orange juice and liqueur and marinate for 1 hour.

Preheat oven to 375°F.

Lightly butter an 8-by-12-inch baking dish. Punch dough down and shape into a ball. Roll it out on a lightly floured board until it is roughly the size of the baking dish. Place in dish and spread with your fingers to cover the entire bottom. Drain pears and distribute over dough, overlapping wedges attractively. Drain raisins and sprinkle, along with pine nuts, over the pears and between the rows. Bake 30 to 45 minutes, until crust is cooked and pears are golden brown. Serve at room temperature.

Serves 8 to 10.

VEGETARIAN

YOU NEED A SOFT PEAR FOR THIS NOT-TOO-SWEET PASTRY. COMICES AND ANJOUS ARE GOOD CHOICES. IT CAN ALSO BE MADE WITH APPLES, AND IN THE SUMMERTIME WITH STRAWBERRIES OR APRICOTS.

cranberry apple roll:
rulet s klyukvoi

PASTRY

3/4 cup butter, at room temperature

6 ounces cream cheese, at room temperature

1 egg yolk

1-1/2 cups flour

1/4 teaspoon salt

FILLING

1 cup cranberries

1/2 cup sugar

2 tablespoons honey

1 tablespoon water

grated peel of 1 lemon

2 tablespoons flour

1/4 teaspoon cinnamon

2 large tart apples, pared, cored, and chopped fine

1 egg yolk, beaten

Cream butter and cream cheese together in a medium bowl. Beat in egg yolk. With your hands, work flour and salt into butter mixture to make a soft dough. Shape into a ball, wrap in waxed paper, and chill at least 30 minutes.

Place cranberries, sugar, honey, water, lemon peel, flour, and cinnamon in a heavy saucepan. Bring to a boil and cook, stirring, about 10 minutes or until cranberries burst. Remove from heat and stir in apples.

Roll dough out and trim it to a 9-by-18-inch rectangle. Leaving a 3-inch strip down the center, cut strips about 1-1/2 inches wide, radiating out from the center down both sides of the dough. A fluted pastry cutter makes a nice design. You should end up with a 3-inch-wide center strip and approximately 12 ribbons of dough on either side.

Spread filling along center strip. Then, alternating sides, fold in the strips at an angle, each one overlapping the next, so that the filling is completely covered. Transfer the roll to a greased baking sheet, using two spatulas. Brush with beaten egg yolk.

Bake approximately 1 hour at 375°F. Cover with foil toward the end so that it doesn't brown too much. Transfer the roll to a rack while still slightly warm. Serve at room temperature.

Serves 8 to 10.

VEGETARIAN

A NICE ADDITION TO A HOLIDAY BUFFET, THIS RUSSIAN BRAIDED PASTRY COMBINES A TART FRUIT FILLING WITH A RICH CRUST. THE PASTRY CAN ALSO BE USED FOR PIROSHKI.

nocciolette

1/2 cup butter, at room temperature

2/3 cup powdered sugar, divided

1 cup flour

1/2 cup shelled hazelnuts, toasted, skinned (preferably), and coarsely ground

1-1/2 tablespoons honey

Preheat oven to 350°F.

Grease a baking sheet. Cream butter with 1/3 cup of the powdered sugar in large bowl until light and fluffy. Add flour, nuts, and honey and beat until smooth.

With lightly floured hands, form dough into 1/2-inch balls and space them 1 inch apart on baking sheet.

Bake until firm, about 15 to 20 minutes. Transfer to rack until cool enough to handle and then roll in the remaining powdered sugar. Store in an airtight container.

Makes 2-1/2 dozen.

VEGETARIAN

ON MY FIRST TRIP TO ITALY, AT AGE 7, I FELL IN LOVE WITH HAZELNUT ICE CREAM. MUCH LATER I LEARNED TO MAKE THESE WONDERFUL LITTLE COOKIES. THEY ARE MORE REFINED IF YOU SKIN THE NUTS, BUT THEY ARE STILL GREAT AND A LOT FASTER IF YOU DON'T, PROVIDED THE NUTS ARE FRESH; THE SKIN GETS BITTER ON NUTS THAT HAVE BEEN AROUND TOO LONG.

carrot torte

3 cups grated carrots

9 tablespoons sugar

4 eggs, separated

2 cups lightly roasted hazelnuts or almonds, ground

1/4 teaspoon allspice

2 teaspoons Marsala (optional)

whipped cream (optional)

Preheat oven to 275°F.

Combine sugar and egg yolks and beat until thickened. Stir in carrots, hazelnuts or almonds, allspice, and Marsala (if used).

Beat egg whites until stiff and fold gently into carrot-nut mixture. Pour gently into a buttered 9-inch pie pan, smooth top, and bake for 1 hour. Serve lukewarm, possibly with Marsala-flavored whipped cream.

Serves 6.

VEGETARIAN, GLUTEN-FREE

ITALIANS MAKE THIS FLOURLESS CAKE WITH ALMONDS. I LIKE IT WITH HAZELNUTS. THE FINER YOU GRATE THE CARROTS, THE MORE DELICATE THE RESULT WILL BE. THE CARROTS FOR THIS RECIPE CAN BE UGLY, BUT THEY MUST BE SWEET; DON'T USE CORKY OLD ONES.

dried fruit tart with pine nuts

PASTRY

2-1/2 cups unbleached flour

1/4 cup sugar

pinch of salt

6 tablespoons unsalted butter

2 large eggs, slightly beaten

1 tablespoon lemon juice

2 tablespoons water

FILLING

15 large prunes

25 dried apricots

3 tablespoons butter

grated rind of 1 lemon

5 tablespoons apricot jam

1-1/4 cups pine nuts

1 egg yolk, beaten

1 tablespoon water

Combine flour, sugar, and salt in a medium bowl. Add butter in small pieces and combine until mixture is crumbly. Add eggs, lemon juice, and water and mix together. The butter will still be a bit lumpy. Turn dough onto a lightly floured surface and knead lightly, just until butter is incorporated into flour. Roll dough into a ball, wrap with waxed paper, and chill at least 1 hour.

Soak prunes and apricots for at least 6 hours in water to cover. Drain and squeeze out excess water. Pit prunes, chop fine, and combine with whole apricots. Blend butter with lemon rind and set aside.

Preheat oven to 350°F and butter a 10-inch pie pan. Reserve a small piece of dough (about 1/5 of the total) and roll out the rest about 1/8-inch thick. Line bottom and sides of pan with dough, allowing extra to drape over the sides. Pierce dough several times with a fork. Spread jam evenly over the surface. (If jam is very thick, dilute with a tablespoon of water.) Distribute chopped fruit over jam, dot with butter and lemon rind, and sprinkle pine nuts over the top. Roll out remaining dough, cut into 1/2-inch-wide strips, and make a lattice crust.

Combine egg yolk and water and brush mixture over top of dough. Bake until crust is golden and pine nuts are brown, about 40 minutes. Serve at room temperature.

Serves 6 to 8.

VEGETARIAN

THE CONCENTRATED FLAVORS GIVE THIS PROVENÇAL DESSERT A REAL IMPACT.
JUST A DELICIOUS SLIVER IS ENOUGH. THE SWEETNESS OF THE DRIED FRUIT MEANS YOU NEED
NO SUGAR BEYOND WHAT'S IN THE JAM. THIS RECIPE IS FROM MEDITERRANEAN HARVEST.
I LIKE TO LEAVE THE APRICOTS WHOLE, FOR LOOKS.

apple applesauce pie

1-3/4 cups unbleached flour

1/4 teaspoon baking powder

1 tablespoon sugar

1/3 cup butter or butter and margarine mixture

FILLING

2-1/2 to 3 cups apples, peeled, cored, and thinly sliced

2 tablespoons flour

1/2 teaspoon salt

3/4 cup sugar

1/2 cup unsweetened yogurt

1/2 cup applesauce

1 egg, lightly beaten

1/2 teaspoon vanilla

Preheat oven to 375°F.

Sift flour, baking powder, and sugar into a bowl. Add shortening, cut into small pieces, and blend with a fork or your fingers until it resembles coarse cornmeal. Press mixture into a pie pan and bake 10 minutes at 400°F. Remove from oven and cool before filling.

Place apples in pie shell. Combine flour, salt, and sugar in a medium bowl. Add yogurt, applesauce, egg, and vanilla and mix well. Pour over apples and bake for about 30 minutes or until mixture has set.

Serves 6.

VEGETARIAN

ONE DAY I SET OUT TO MAKE MRS. ANDERSON'S SOUR CREAM APPLE PIE (THE RECIPE IS IN LILA GAULT'S *NORTHWEST COOKBOOK* AND IT'S GREAT) AND FOUND I DIDN'T HAVE ANY SOUR CREAM. THE FOLLOWING IMPROVISATION IS A BIT EASIER ON THE ARTERIES, AND IT GOT RAVES. I HATE MAKING PIE CRUST SO I USE A PAT-IN-THE-PAN KUCHEN PASTRY WHENEVER POSSIBLE.

PUMPKIN PIE

One Thanksgiving not long after I was married, I brought pumpkin pie to Thanksgiving dinner at my in-laws. I was proud, probably long-windedly proud, to tell the table that we had grown the pumpkin, hand milked the cow for the milk and churned the butter, rendered the lard from our own hogs, and gathered the eggs from chickens we had raised ourselves. We baked it in the oven of our wood cook stove, after cutting, splitting and hauling the wood. I waited for applause. My mother-in-law, a tiny, regal woman, put down her cigarette, widened her big brown eyes and said, in the Alabama accent she could never quite extinguish, though she tried—"Oh my Gawd. Why?" Not everyone thrills to symbolic self-sufficiency. But I *liked* doing all those things. And it was a very good pie.

Not many cooks are in a position to go to that extreme, but making pie from fresh pumpkin is well within reach. Any favorite pie recipe is fine. The trick is to minimize the hassle of preparing the purée. A good-sized pumpkin will make several pies. I freeze the purée in pie-sized portions, making it—after the initial labor—as convenient as canned. These instructions also apply to squash pies. As specialty squashes proliferate, the possibilities for variations in pie flavor also expand. You could have a pie tasting with several different varieties. Pumpkin pie recipes also make perfectly good custards. Just heat the oven heat to 350°F and set the custard dish in a pan of hot water.

PREPARING THE PURÉE

Cut pumpkin in half and scrape out seeds and strings. (I am usually too impatient to clean and toast seeds for a snack, but my daughter likes that job.) Place the halves cut side down on a cookie sheet or in a roasting pan. Don't use a rimless baking sheet because the pumpkins will ooze as they cook. Bake at 325°F until pumpkin is squishy when poked. It should be really soft but not beginning to burn.

Remove from oven and let cool a bit. Pour off the collected pumpkin juice and save. Peel the pumpkin, or scoop out the insides with a spoon. Purée the flesh bit by bit in a blender, adding some of the juice whenever needed. Get the mixture really smooth. Measure out a pie's worth of purée and freeze or can the rest. Then you are ready to proceed with your favorite recipe, or with the following one.

olga hemmestad's pumpkin pie

1-1/2 cups half-and-half

1/4 teaspoon maple extract

3/4 cup light brown sugar

1/2 teaspoon salt

1/2 teaspoon cinnamon

1/4 teaspoon nutmeg

1/4 teaspoon ginger

1-1/2 cups pumpkin, cooked and puréed

3 whole eggs, beaten

pastry for single-crust 9-inch pie

Preheat oven to 400°F.

Bring half-and-half to a boil, remove from heat, and add maple extract. Combine all other ingredients and add to the half-and-half. Mix well. Pour into pie shell and bake about 40 minutes.

Serves 6.

VEGETARIAN

YEARS AGO THE BELLINGHAM FARMERS MARKET HAD A PUMPKIN PIE CONTEST.
MRS. HEMMESTAD, AN ENERGETIC TESTIMONY TO THE EXCELLENCE OF
HER OWN COOKING AT AGE 90, WON WITH THIS RECIPE. IT IS NOT HIGHLY SPICED,
WHICH ALLOWS YOU TO APPRECIATE THE SUBTLETIES OF YOUR HOMEGROWN SQUASH.

rutabaga pie

2 medium rutabagas

1 cup light brown sugar

2 tablespoons maple syrup

2 eggs, lightly beaten

1-1/4 cups half-and-half

1/2 teaspoon ginger

1 teaspoon cinnamon

1/2 teaspoon nutmeg

1/2 teaspoon cloves

1/2 teaspoon salt

1 teaspoon vanilla

pastry for single-crust 9-inch pie

Preheat oven to 450°F.

Peel rutabagas and cut into chunks. Cook in a minimum of gently boiling water until soft, 25 to 30 minutes. Drain. Purée rutabagas in a blender. You should have 1-1/2 cups. Add all remaining ingredients and blend until smooth. Pour into pastry shell.

Bake 15 minutes at 450°F, reduce heat to 350°F, and bake another 40 minutes or until mixture is set.

Serves 6.

VEGETARIAN

THIS RECIPE IS FROM MAINE, HOME OF THE GREAT-TASTING LAURENTIAN RUTABAGA.
IF I DIDN'T KNOW WHAT I WAS EATING, I WOULD THINK IT WAS A PUMPKIN PIE WITH AN EXTRA
PINCH OF CLOVES. IT'S REALLY GOOD, AND RUTABAGAS ARE CERTAINLY MORE CONVENIENT
THAN FRESH PUMPKIN FOR PEELING AND PURÉEING. IF YOU GROW YOUR OWN RUTABAGAS,
HARVEST AFTER A FROST AND YOUR PIE WILL BE THAT MUCH BETTER.

apple pastila

3 large, tart apples

1 teaspoon fresh lemon juice

1 cup sugar

1/4 teaspoon almond extract

1/4 teaspoon cinnamon

2 egg whites

Peel, halve, and core apples, and steam over boiling water until tender. Purée apples and pour into a large bowl. Stir in lemon juice, sugar, almond extract, and cinnamon.

Beat egg whites until stiff but not dry. Stir into apple mixture. Beat at high speed for at least 5 minutes, or for 10 to 15 minutes by hand.

Preheat oven to 150°F.

Spread a sheet of bakers parchment on a baking sheet. Drop the apple foam by tablespoonfuls onto the parchment.

Bake about 6 hours, until confections are dry to the touch. Transfer to a wire rack to cool. Keep in a tightly closed container until just before serving.

Makes about 5 dozen.

VEGETARIAN, GLUTEN-FREE

THIS 19TH-CENTURY RUSSIAN confection smells heavenly while it is cooking. (Actually, it's more a drying than a cooking—very low and very slow.) The meringues will be alarmingly chewy when they come out of the oven but will turn crisp and light as they dry.

carrot halvah

3 cups milk

1/2 cup brown sugar (Mexican canela cones, or the unrefined brown sugar such as succanat now sold in some supermarkets are the closest to Indian sugar)

2 cups coarsely grated carrots (3 or 4 medium)

10 pods cardamom (about 1/2 teaspoon ground)

1/2 cup unsalted butter or ghee (*see page 236*)

1/2 cup almonds, chopped

1/2 cup raisins

1/4 teaspoon mace

2 tablespoons honey

Bring milk to a boil in a heavy saucepan. Add brown sugar and carrots. Return to boil, reduce to just below the boiling point, and cook, uncovered, for 45 minutes, stirring often to keep carrots from sticking. The liquid should reduce by at least half and the mixture should be quite thick.

Take cardamom seeds from their pods and crush them with a rolling pin or a mortar and pestle. Melt butter in a large frying pan and sauté almonds and raisins for 2 minutes. Add cardamom and mace to frying pan and stir well. Stir in honey and cook another minute. Pour in milk and carrot mixture and bring to a boil. Cook, stirring constantly, until halvah begins to stiffen and pull away from the sides of the pan.

Remove from heat, spoon into a shallow, flat dish, and smooth top. Let cool before serving. Refrigerate for an hour if you what to cut the halvah into the traditional diamond shapes.

Serves 8.

VEGETARIAN, GLUTEN-FREE

INDIAN COOKING INCLUDES AN ARRAY OF MILK-BASED SWEETS, MANY OF THEM THE PROVINCE OF PROFESSIONAL CANDY COOKS. HOWEVER, THIS SIMPLE VERSION IS GENERALLY MADE AT HOME. IT IS MUCH MOISTER THAN THE GROUND-SESAME HALVAH SOLD IN THIS COUNTRY, AND IT DOES NOT KEEP AS LONG. (THE LATTER HAS NOT BEEN A PROBLEM AT OUR HOUSE.) WHOLE CARDAMOM AND UNSALTED BUTTER DO MAKE A DIFFERENCE IN THIS RECIPE.

pears in syrup

6 Seckel or Bosc pears

2/3 cup sugar

up to 1 bottle of dry red wine

1-by-3-inch section orange rind

1 stick cinnamon

6 whole cloves

three 1/4-inch slices fresh ginger

4 threads saffron (optional)

whipped cream or custard sauce

Peel pears, leaving stems on. Stand them upright in a deep, narrow earthenware or enamel casserole with cover. Add sugar and enough wine to cover halfway. Tie orange rind, cinnamon, cloves, ginger, and saffron (if used) in cheesecloth and add to casserole. Add enough water to cover pears.

Cover casserole and bake at 250°F for 5 to 7 hours, basting pears occasionally as liquid cooks down. Bake until liquid is a rich syrup and pears are completely tender but not falling apart. Cool in syrup. Remove spice bag and serve pears with whipped cream or custard sauce.

Serves 6.

VEGETARIAN, GLUTEN-FREE

THERE ARE LOTS OF GOOD RECIPES FOR POACHED PEARS. THIS IS ONE OF THE OLDEST, TRACING ITS LINEAGE TO A MEDIEVAL DISH THAT USED VINEGAR RATHER THAN WINE. IT'S A GOOD USE FOR BOSCS OR SECKEL PEARS, AN HEIRLOOM VARIETY THAT SHOWS UP IN MANY OLD ORCHARDS AND SOMETIMES IN STORES. SECKELS ARE SMALL AND BROWNISH GREEN, WITH LONG NECKS. THE ONES IN SUMAS WERE READY IN OCTOBER AND KEPT ABOUT A MONTH. THEY TASTE QUITE A LOT LIKE ASIAN PEARS, BEING HARD AND NOT PARTICULARLY SWEET. I DON'T CARE FOR THEM FRESH, BUT THEY ARE GREAT FOR COOKING. THIS RECIPE IS VEGAN IF YOU SKIP THE TOPPING.

cranberry macaroon cream

1 cup whipping cream

1/2 cup sugar

6 ounces cranberries (half a package)

4 teaspoons chopped fresh mint leaves

1-1/2 cups crumbled coconut macaroons

⊰⊱ cook's note

Cranberries are easier to chop when partly frozen.

Whip cream until stiff, adding sugar gradually. Chop cranberries by hand or in blender. Stir cranberries and mint leaves into whipped cream. Add macaroons, stir carefully, and chill at least an hour.

Serves 4.

VEGETARIAN

TART CRANBERRIES AND RICH MACAROONS ARE A SURPRISING COMBINATION.
I MAKE THIS IN NOVEMBER WITH THE LAST MINT OF THE SEASON.
CRANBERRIES ARE EASIER TO CHOP WHEN THEY ARE PARTLY FROZEN.

hazelnut pie

2 eggs

1/2 cup sugar

pinch salt

3/4 cup dark corn syrup

1 tablespoon melted butter

1/2 teaspoon vanilla

2 cups finely chopped roasted hazelnuts

pastry for single-crust 9-inch pie

Preheat oven to 325°F.

Beat eggs in medium bowl. Add in order: sugar, salt, corn syrup, melted butter, and vanilla. Mix until blended and then stir in hazelnuts. Pour into pie shell and bake 50 to 60 minutes.

Makes one 9-inch pie.

VEGETARIAN

THIS IS THE NORTHWEST ANSWER TO PECAN PIE. THE RECIPE COMES FROM HOLMQUIST HAZELNUTS,
A SMALL ORCHARD IN NORTHWEST WASHINGTON. I CAN HARDLY EMPHASIZE HOW GOOD IT IS.

winter fruit bars

2 cups fruit (see below)

1/4 cup soft butter

1/3 cup brown sugar

3/4 cup whole wheat flour

3/4 teaspoon salt

1/2 teaspoon baking powder

1/2 to 1 teaspoon cinnamon, to taste

2/3 cup oatmeal

3-4 tablespoons oat bran

3-4 tablespoons olive oil

Prepare fruit; preheat oven to 350°F.

In a 9-inch pie plate, mix butter and brown sugar.

When sugar is dissolved and the mix is smooth, add remaining ingredients.

Mix with hands or with a spoon; it's easiest to sprinkle the olive oil over the mixture until it becomes crumbly. Pat about two-thirds of the mixture firmly and evenly over the bottom of the pie plate, reserving the rest for topping. Add fruit, sprinkle remaining mixture over the top, and bake 30 minutes.

Makes one 9-inch pan.

VEGETARIAN

MY FRIEND AND NEIGHBOR CAROLYN DALE INVENTED THIS VERSATILE RECIPE, AND I'LL LET HER DESCRIBE IT. SHE IS A TERRIFIC COOK. "INSPIRED BY HARVEST BARS AND DATE BARS, THIS RECIPE ADAPTS TO A RANGE OF FRESH AND DRIED FRUITS. DATES ARE GREAT, ALONE. DRIED FRUIT SHOULD BE RECONSTITUTED UNTIL MOIST: PLACE ABOUT TWO CUPS IN A SMALL SAUCEPAN AND JUST COVER WITH WATER. SIMMER FOR FIVE MINUTES OR SO AND DRAIN OFF WATER THAT HAS NOT BEEN ABSORBED. OR, A LAYER OF DRIED FRUIT CAN BE TOPPED BY A LAYER OF FRESH FRUIT, SUCH AS APRICOTS. DURING THE WINTER, I LOVE USING RIPENED PEARS OVER A COMBINATION OF DRIED PLUMS, RAISINS AND APRICOTS SIMMERED IN WATER WITH A TOUCH OF BRANDY AND LEMON PEEL. THESE ARE QUICK TO MAKE AND ARE GREAT TO SERVE ANY TIME OF DAY, OR EVEN AS DESSERT."

quince sorbet

1 cup water

2 cups sugar

2 large (apple-sized) quinces

half an egg white, lightly beaten

Boil water and sugar to make a thin syrup. Remove from heat and let cool. Peel and seed quinces, slice, and place in saucepan with just enough water to keep from burning. Cook, covered, until soft. Remove from heat and purée. You should have 1-1/2 cups. Cool, and then add 2/3 cup of the syrup and the egg white. Process in an ice cream maker.

Makes 1 pint.

VEGETARIAN, GLUTEN-FREE

ROBIN SAUNDERS, CO-OWNER OF LE GOURMAND IN SEATTLE, PROVIDED THE RECIPE FOR THIS TANGY GOLDEN SORBET.

rose pear granita

1 quart pear juice

1/2 cup rose hips, cut in half and seeded

Pour juice into a saucepan, add rose hips, and simmer, covered, until liquid is reduced by half. Put through a food mill and pour into a shallow pan. Freeze. Stir when mixture starts to get slushy and return to freezer until time to serve.

Makes 1 pint.

VEGAN, GLUTEN-FREE

NO SPECIAL EQUIPMENT IS REQUIRED FOR THIS SIMPLE ICE FROM LE GOURMAND.
THE ROSE HIPS GIVE THE CRYSTALS A BIT OF TARTNESS AND A GORGEOUS RED-GOLD TINT.
THIS MAKES A GOOD DIGESTIVE AS WELL AS A DECEPTIVELY SIMPLE DESSERT.

hazelnut roca

1/2 pound unsalted butter

1 cup sugar

1/2 cup chopped hazelnuts

1/2 cup ground hazelnuts

one 6-ounce package semisweet chocolate chips

Melt butter over high heat in a cast-iron skillet or other heavy, shallow pan. Add sugar, bit by bit, as butter is melting. Stir constantly but gently. When sugar starts to change color, add chopped hazelnuts. Stir and test for hard-crack stage in cold water. Pour into a shallow pan and cool. (Any "runoff" of melted butter from the cooling candy can be poured off and saved to use in other baking. It has a wonderful flavor.) Score the candy lightly before it's fully cool so it will be easier to break into tidy pieces.

Melt chocolate chips in a double boiler over simmering water. Stir in ground hazelnuts and spread chocolate mixture over the cooled candy. When cold, break into pieces.

Makes 30 1-by-2-inch candies.

VEGETARIAN

THE YEAR I MADE THIS WITH NUTS FROM OUR OWN TREES AND BUTTER FROM OUR OWN COW; I FELT I HAD REACHED THE PINNACLE OF COUNTRY LIVING. NOW I'M BACK TO STORE-BOUGHT INGREDIENTS, BUT THIS CANDY IS STILL A FAVORITE ADDITION TO THE CHRISTMAS COOKIE PLATE.

cranberry lemon cookies

1 cup of butter, softened

1 cup white sugar

1/2 cup brown sugar (I use succanat)

2 eggs

1 cup milk (I use unsweetened soy milk)

1/4 cup fresh lemon juice

2 teaspoons vanilla extract

4 cups all-purpose flour

4 teaspoons baking powder

1 teaspoon salt

2 tablespoons lemon rind, peeled and chopped

1-1/2 cups fresh or frozen cranberries

Preheat oven to 350°F.

Cream butter and sugar until light. Add eggs, milk, lemon juice and vanilla and beat until smooth. In another bowl, combine flour, baking powder and salt. Stir in dry ingredients. Then add cranberries and lemon rind and mix well.

Refrigerate dough for at least an hour to firm. Drop by spoonfuls onto a prepared cookie sheet and bake until tops are firm and bottoms are light brown. Cool before serving.

Makes 3 dozen.

VEGETARIAN

JUST TART ENOUGH, AND VERY PRETTY WITH THEIR STUDDING OF CRANBERRIES. I MAKE THEM WITH MEYER LEMONS FROM MY CONTAINER TREE, SO THEY HAVE A BIT MORE LOCAVORE CRED. FRESH LEMON RIND CAN BE AN ISSUE FOR HEALTH-CONSCIOUS COOKS WHO CAN'T GROW THEIR OWN. ORGANIC LEMONS ARE EXPENSIVE, AND NON-ORGANIC ONES TEND TO BE HEAVILY SPRAYED. MY SOLUTION WHEN I'M OUT OF HOME-GROWN IS TO BUY ORGANIC AND FREEZE THE SQUEEZED OUT REMAINDERS. WHEN I NEED FRESH RIND, I JUST TAKE THE BAGGY OUT OF THE FREEZER AND PEEL THE RINDS RIGHT THERE. THE TASTE DOESN'T CHANGE, AND AS A BONUS, THE FROZEN RINDS ARE MUCH EASIER TO PEEL OR GRATE.

maple parsnip drop cookies

1-1/2 cups maple syrup

3/4 cup peeled, grated parsnip

1/2 cup canola oil

1 egg, beaten

1 teaspoon salt

1-1/2 cups flour, sifted

2 teaspoons baking powder

1/4 cup milk

1-1/2 cups rolled oats

1/2 cup chopped nuts

Preheat oven to 350°F.

Simmer the maple syrup and parsnips in a medium saucepan until parsnips are soft. Remove mixture from heat and let cool. Beat the oil and maple syrup in a medium bowl until light. Add the egg and mix thoroughly.

In a separate bowl, sift together the flour, salt, and baking powder. Add the dry ingredients to the maple syrup mixture in two parts, alternating with the milk. Stir well.

Then stir in raisins, nuts, and rolled oats.

Drop by spoonfuls on prepared cookie sheet. Bake at 350° for about 15 minutes.

Makes 3 dozen.

VEGETARIAN

I'VE READ SOME ENGLISH WWII-ERA RECIPES FOR MARMALADE MADE WITH MATCHSTICKS OF PARSNIPS STANDING IN FOR THE UNOBTAINABLE ORANGES. ALTHOUGH I LIKED THE IMAGE OF A LEGION OF BRITISH COOKS, UNSTIFFENING THEIR UPPER LIPS JUST ENOUGH TO SAY, "AH WELL, MUSTN'T GRUMBLE," IT DIDN'T ACTUALLY SOUND VERY TASTY. THESE PARSNIP COOKIES, ON THE OTHER HAND, TASTE WAY BETTER THAN THEY MAY SOUND. I TOOK A BATCH TO SCHOOL, WHERE THEY PASSED THE TEENAGER TEST, MEANING THAT THEY DON'T TASTE TOO WEIRD OR TOO HEALTHY FOR THE AVERAGE 16-YEAR-OLD. IF YOU'VE GOT THE CHEAPER, DARKER, B-GRADE SYRUP, THIS IS THE PLACE TO USE IT. MOLASSES WOULD WORK TOO.

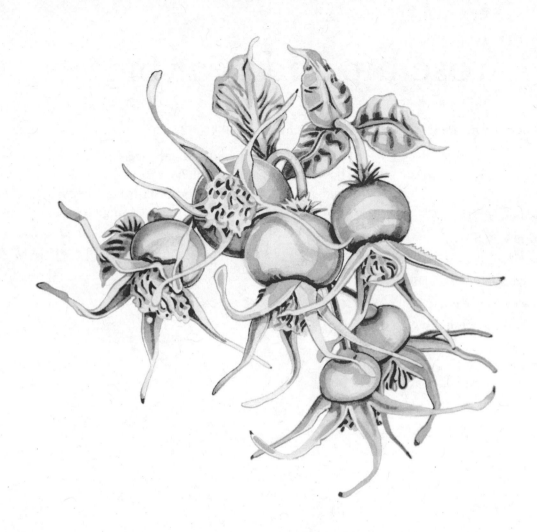

rosehips

· · · · · · · · · · · · · · · · · · · ·

rose hip and pear pie

1-1/2 tablespoons cornstarch

1 cup sugar

2 eggs

1/2 cup milk

3/4 cup agave syrup

1/4 teaspoon salt

1 teaspoon vanilla

2 or 3 cups halved, seeded rosehips

1-1/2 cups peeled, sliced pear

pastry for double-crust 9-inch pie

Preheat oven to 350°F.

Mix the cornstarch and sugar together in a medium bowl. In a separate bowl, beat the eggs, milk, syrup, salt, and vanilla. Add the liquid mixture to the cornstarch and sugar and mix thoroughly. Arrange the pear slices on the pie shell, place the rose hips on top, and pour the liquid mixture over the top. Top with a lattice crust. Bake 35 to 40 minutes or until set.

Makes one 9-inch pie.

VEGETARIAN

THIS IS ADAPTED FROM A RECIPE BY MARIAN GLENZ, WHO FOR MANY YEARS RAN THE STORE IN THE ALASKAN FISHING VILLAGE OF MEYERS CHUCK, NEAR KETCHIKAN, AND WROTE A BOOK ABOUT HER LIFE THERE. HAVING MORE CHOICES OF INGREDIENTS TO WORK WITH, I REPLACED THE CORN SYRUP AND ADDED PEARS, BECAUSE AS SHE NOTED, COOKED ROSE HIPS ON THEIR OWN CAN BE A BIT "BLAH." HER ORIGINAL RECIPE WAS ONE I CHOSE FOR THE TERRITORIAL SEED COMPANY COOKBOOK. WHOLE CRANBERRIES COULD BE SUBSTITUTED FOR THE ROSE HIPS.

sweet potato
and pear muffins

1 cup whole wheat flour

1 cup all purpose flour

1/3 cup brown sugar or succanat

2-1/2 teaspoons baking powder

1/2 teaspoon cinnamon

1/4 teaspoon ground coriander or
cardamom (both flavors are great
with pears)

1/2 teaspoon salt

1 cup milk (I use 1 percent)

1 large egg

1 tablespoon canola oil

1 cup grated raw sweet potato

1/2 cup finely chopped dried pears

Preheat oven to 375°F.

Prepare 12 muffin cups with oil, cooking spray, or paper cups.

Combine flours, sugar, baking powder, spices, and salt in a medium mixing bowl.

In a separate bowl, combine milk, egg, and oil and beat lightly.

Make a well in the center of the dry ingredients, pour in the liquids, and stir until just combined. A few lumps are OK.

Fold in the sweet potatoes and pears.

Fill muffin cups 2/3 full. Bake 18 to 20 minutes, until springy.

Makes 12 muffins.

VEGETARIAN

THESE ARE NOT YOUR FLUFFY MUFFINS. THEY ARE DENSE AND CHEWY, BUT NOT GRIMLY HEALTHY; THEY TASTE REALLY GOOD. PEARS ARE AMONG THE EASIEST FRUIT TO DRY, WHICH IS A GOOD THING BECAUSE THEY TEND TO RIPEN IN A RUSH. THEY ARE ALSO VERY SWEET, SO YOU CAN CUT BACK ON OTHER SUGAR. AS WITH ALL MUFFINS, YOU WANT TO AVOID ACTIVATING THE GLUTEN IN THE FLOUR, SO DON'T OVER-MIX THE BATTER. I ADAPTED THE RECIPE FROM RELISHMAG.COM.

pumkin coffee cake

2 cups flour

1/2 cup granulated sugar

1-1/2 teaspoons baking powder

1 teaspoon salt, divided

6 tablespoons butter

3 eggs

1/3 cup milk

2-1/4 cups pumpkin purée

1 teaspoon cinnamon

1/2 teaspoon ground allspice

1/2 teaspoon ground ginger

1/2 cup plus 2 tablespoons light brown sugar, divided

1/2 teaspoon freshly grated nutmeg

Preheat oven to 350°F.

Grease a 9-by-13-inch baking dish. Combine flour, white sugar, baking powder, and 1/2 teaspoon of the salt in a large bowl. Blend thoroughly. Cut in butter until mixture is crumbly. Take out half the mixture and put it in another bowl.

Beat 1 egg and milk in a separate bowl. Pour over one portion of the pastry mixture and toss with fork until moistened. Pat gently into baking dish and bake for 10 minutes. Remove from oven.

In yet another bowl, combine pumpkin purée, remaining 2 eggs, cinnamon, allspice, ginger, and remaining 1/2 teaspoon salt. Add 1/4 cup of the brown sugar and blend well. Pour mixture over the cooked crust. Stir nutmeg and remaining brown sugar into reserved flour mixture and toss with fork. Sprinkle over filling. Bake for 30 to 40 minutes or until filling is set. Cool until filling is firm.

Makes one 9-by-13-inch cake.

VEGETARIAN

PUMPKIN PIE FILLING GOES ON TOP OF A LAYER OF SWEET BATTER, WITH STREUSEL TOPPING OVER ALL. THIS QUICK SWEET IS SIMPLE TO MAKE, BUT IT DOES USE LOTS OF BOWLS.

nutella pudding cake

3/4 cup agave syrup

2-1/2 cups peeled, chopped beets

1/2 cup water

4 eggs

1/2 cup light oil (canola or grapeseed)

1 tablespoon vanilla extract

1/2 cup fine-ground hazelnuts (I use a coffee grinder)

1/2 cup cocoa powder

1/2 teaspoon salt

Preheat oven to 350°F.

Pour the syrup into a medium saucepan, add the chopped beets, and bring to a boil. Cover and simmer until beets are soft, about 30 minutes. Purée the mixture until as smooth as you can get it. Mix in the eggs, oil, and vanilla. Mix the nuts, cocoa, and salt into a large bowl, add the beet mixture, and stir thoroughly.

Pour batter into a greased, 9-inch cake pan and bake until a knife in the center comes out clean, 30–40 minutes. The sides will puff up a bit, and the center will stay moist.

Cool before serving. I sift a little powdered sugar on top for contrast.

Makes one 9-inch cake.

VEGETARIAN, GLUTEN-FREE

RICH, DARK, MOIST, NON-DAIRY, AND GLUTEN-FREE, THIS TREAT DELIVERS ONE OF MY FAVORITE FLAVOR COMBOS—CHOCOLATE AND HAZELNUT—WITH THE HIDDEN SURPRISE OF BEETS, WHICH PROVIDE THE TEXTURE AND TINT OF AN OLD-FASHIONED VELVET CAKE. IT IS A FINE USE FOR THE GREAT BIG, OVERWINTERED BEET VARIETIES, AND A REMINDER THAT SUGAR BEETS USED TO BE A MAJOR CROP IN THE PACIFIC NORTHWEST. IT'S MODIFIED FROM A RECIPE BY ELANA AMSTERDAM, AUTHOR OF *THE GLUTEN-FREE, ALMOND FLOUR COOKBOOK* AND THE ELANA'S PANTRY BLOG, ELANASPANTRY.COM. ELANA'S MOTTO IS "SIMPLIFY, SATISFY." IN THIS CASE YOU COULD PROBABLY ADD, "SEDUCE," RICH AND SILKY AS IT IS.

carrot ginger hazelnut cake

3/4 cup agave syrup

3 cups peeled, chopped carrots

3 eggs, beaten

1/2 cup light oil (canola or grapeseed)

1 tablespoon vanilla extract

1/2 cup fine-ground hazelnuts (I use a coffee grinder)

1/2 cup flour

1/4 cup candied ginger, chopped

1 teaspoon ground ginger

1/2 teaspoon salt

Preheat oven to 350°F.

Pour the syrup into a medium saucepan, add the chopped carrots, and bring to a boil. Cover and simmer until carrots are soft, about 20 minutes. Purée the mixture until it's as smooth as you can get it. Mix in the eggs, oil, and vanilla. Mix the nuts, flour, ginger, and salt, into a large bowl, add the carrot purée and the chopped ginger, and stir thoroughly.

Pour batter into a greased, 9-inch cake pan and bake until a knife in the center comes out clean, 30–40 minutes. The center will stay moist.

Cool before serving. I like it plain, but a bit of whipped cream or crème fraiche is always welcome.

Makes one 9-inch cake.

VEGETARIAN

THIS RECIPE CONTAINS WHEAT FLOUR, BUT IT CERTAINLY COULD BE GLUTEN-FREE BY USING MORE GROUND HAZELNUTS OR CHESTNUT FLOUR. RATTY-LOOKING, SWEET-TASTING WINTER CARROTS ARE IDEAL.

pumpkin and prune pie

1 pound pumpkin, peeled and chopped into 1-inch sections, or 1-1/2 cups puréed pumpkin

3 tablespoons butter

20 prunes, pitted and soaked until soft

1 cup half-and-half

4 tablespoons sugar

pastry for double-crust 9-inch pie

Preheat oven to 400°F.

Melt butter in a medium skillet and cook pumpkin gently until it is reduced to a purée. Remove from heat, add prunes, half-and-half, and sugar and mix well.

Line pie dish with bottom crust, put in filling, and cover with top crust. Bake 10 minutes at 400°F. Lower heat to 350°F and bake another 30 minutes.

Serves 6.

VEGETARIAN

ELIZABETH DAVID HELPED INTRODUCE ENGLISH-SPEAKING COOKS TO CONTINENTAL CUISINES, INCLUDING RECIPES FOR THAT NEW WORLD TRANSPLANT, THE PUMPKIN. YOU MAY NOT RECOGNIZE YOUR OLD THANKSGIVING STANDBY WITHOUT ITS FAMILIAR SPICES. A SWEET WINTER SQUASH SUCH AS DELICATA CAN BE SUBSTITUTED FOR PUMPKIN, AND IT SHOULD BE IF YOUR ONLY PUMPKIN IS A JACK-O'-LANTERN GIANT. IF I DIDN'T GROW MY OWN PIE PUMPKINS, I WOULDN'T BOTHER WITH FRESH PUMPKIN ANYWAY; CANNED PURÉE IS JUST FINE FOR PIES AND CUSTARDS, AND THE DENSE WINTER SQUASHES HAVE SUPERIOR FLAVOR FOR MOST USES.

spinach tart

1 cup milk or half-and-half

2 eggs

1/3 cup sugar

2 cups cooked spinach, drained

grated rind of 1 small lemon

1 teaspoon vanilla

1/2 cup apricot jam

pastry for single-crust 9-inch pie, plus extra for lattice if desired

Preheat oven to 450°F.

Blend milk or half-and-half, eggs, and sugar in top of a double broiler. Cook slowly, stirring constantly, until mixture thickens enough to coat the spoon. Chop spinach, press dry, and stir into custard with lemon rind and vanilla. Melt jam in a small saucepan over low heat.

Spoon half of spinach mixture into pie shell. Cover with 1/3 cup of the jam, then the rest of the spinach, and then the remainder of the jam. Add a lattice top crust if you wish.

Bake 20 minutes. Serve at room temperature.

Serves 6.

VEGETARIAN

I FIRST TRIED THIS UNUSUAL COMBINATION MANY YEARS AGO AT SEATTLE'S RAISON D'ETRE COFFEEHOUSE. ITS FRESH TASTE MAKES A NICE CHANGE FOR THE WINTER ROUND OF PUMPKIN AND APPLE PIES. SPINACH DESSERTS REPORTEDLY DATE BACK TO THE TIME OF THE RENAISSANCE, WHEN FRENCH AND ENGLISH COOKS BEGAN EXPLORING THE POSSIBILITIES OF THE VEGETABLE, NEWLY ARRIVED FROM SPAIN. A REGIONAL VARIATION IS SORREL PIE, A SPECIALTY OF THE BLASKET ISLANDS OFF THE COAST OF IRELAND.

côte d'azur tart

1/3 cup pine nuts, lightly toasted

1-1/2 cups chopped chard

2 tablespoons currants or raisins, soaked in 3 tablespoons dark rum for 20 minutes

2 eggs, beaten

1/2 cup sugar

1/4 cup grated Parmesan cheese

pinch of black pepper

3 cups peeled, cored, and sliced apples or firm pears

pastry for a double-crust 9-inch pie

Preheat oven to 375°F.

Toast pine nuts lightly in an ungreased skillet over medium heat and set aside.

Bring 1 cup of water to a boil in a medium saucepan, add chard, and cook, covered, over medium heat for 10 minutes. Drain and squeeze out all excess water once chard is cool enough to handle. Combine all remaining ingredients except the apples in a large mixing bowl, then blend in the chard.

Smooth chard mixture evenly across bottom of pie shell and cover with apple slices. Roll out remaining dough and cover pie, pressing to join edges. Prick top crust to let steam escape. Bake for 50 minutes to 1 hour, until crust is browned and filling firm. Cover top crust with foil if it browns before filling is ready. Serve warm or at room temperature.

Serves 6.

VEGETARIAN

If you like the Spinach Tart, you can move on to an even odder combination of Swiss chard, apples, raisins, and Parmesan cheese. This recipe is from *Mediterranean Harvest*, which is a wonderful resource for adventurous cooks.

carrot parsnip custard

4 tablespoons butter

2 cups finely grated carrots

1 cup finely grated parsnips

1/4 cup flour

1 teaspoon salt

1/2 teaspoon ground ginger

3 eggs, lightly beaten

1/3 cup maple syrup

1-1/2 cups half-and-half

Preheat oven to 325°F.

Melt butter in a large saucepan, add carrots and parsnips, and sauté gently for about 5 minutes, until vegetables begin to soften. Remove from heat. Combine flour, salt, and ginger and stir mixture into vegetables. Add eggs, maple syrup, and half-and-half and stir well.

Pour into buttered custard dish and set in pan of boiling water. Water should always be about 1 inch up on sides of dish. Add more boiling water while baking, if necessary. Bake until knife inserted in center comes out clean, about 1-1/2 to 2 hours.

Serves 6.

VEGETARIAN

YOU COULD MAKE THIS WITH 3 CUPS OF CARROTS AND NO PARSNIPS, BUT THE COMBINATION GIVES A NICE BLEND IN BOTH FLAVOR AND COLOR. AFTER YEARS OF FRUSTRATION TRYING TO GET A CUSTARD DISH INTO A PAN OF BOILING WATER WITHOUT BURNING MYSELF OR SPLASHING MY CREATION, I FOUND THE ANSWER. PLACE THE CUSTARD DISH IN A DEEP EMPTY PAN—I USE A SOUP KETTLE—AND THEN STICK A FUNNEL BETWEEN DISH AND KETTLE AND POUR THE BOILING WATER THROUGH IT. MAYBE YOU ALREADY KNEW THAT.

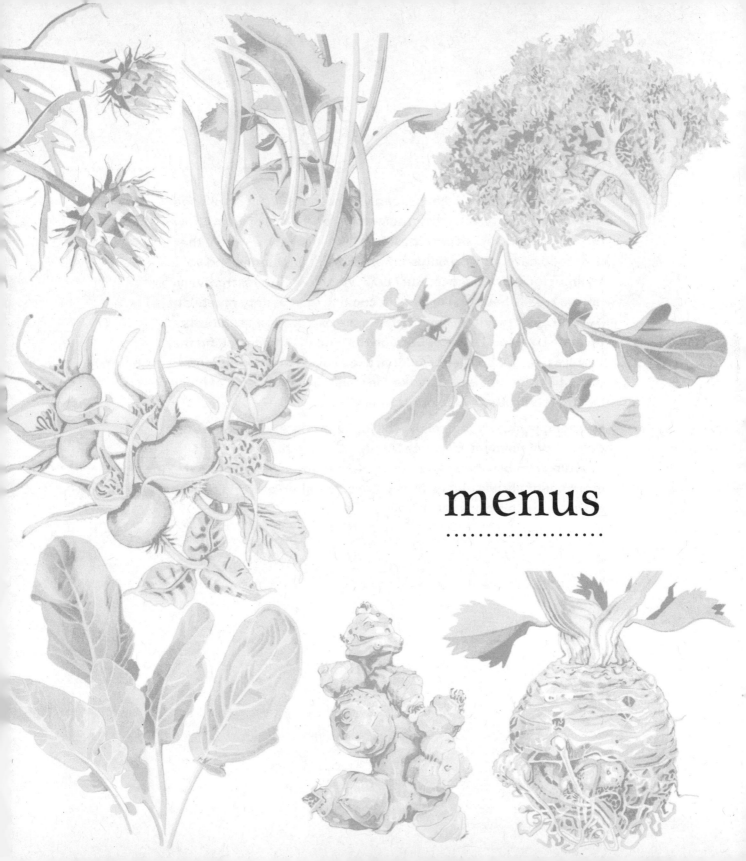

menus

MENUS

A truly seasonal, local diet probably is most easily accomplished by having just a few main ingredients for each time of year. Grow lots of kale and lots of potatoes. Boil them one day, fry them the next, add hazelnuts on Saturday and an egg on Sunday and voila: a winter locavore is made. But I don't want to eat so restrictively unless I really have to. I'm used to cooking for a variety of reasons beyond basic nutrition, among them the exploration of cultures through cuisine. I have cut back on the kind of ethnic cooking that requires a large battery of seldom used spices and condiments, but I still want meals that evoke the traditions and tastes of places I've traveled either in life or in fantasy.

The sample menus that follow call for fresh winter vegetables and do not contain meat, because I figured that might be the most daunting combination of factors for someone who wants to eat more mindfully without giving up the exploration of world cuisines. Dishes from this book are in italics.

eastern european

Beets, cabbage and mushrooms are the foundation of Slavic winter cooking. Sour flavorings—from vinegar, yogurt, lemon, or sauerkraut—show influences of the Central European, Middle Eastern, and Mediterranean cultures that have collided, and sometimes melded, in the Balkans. It's hard to imagine a Slavic meal without soup or a loaf of dense white bread.

Mushroom Ciorba

Polenta Stuffed Cabbage or Russian Vegetable Pie

Roasted Beets

Bread

Walnut Torte

italian

Fresh tomatoes, green beans, zucchini, fresh basil—can we really cook an Italian meal without them? One clue to the answer is that Italy had a vibrant cuisine long before any of those ingredients, except maybe the basil, arrived. And even in the sunniest parts of Sicily, you can't harvest a garden tomato in January. A traditional Italian meal is served course by course rather than all at once, the better to sit and talk long into the night.

Bagna Cauda

Kale Manicotti

Grilled Portabella Mushrooms

Escarole and Cabbage Salad

Nocciolette

indian

· ·

Although Indian food brings to mind vivid summer flavors and
tropical tastes, the subcontinent has a vast range of climate and
topography. High altitudes restrict many areas to cold-tolerant vegetables. I recently read a recipe for a lamb and turnip curry that said
the turnips were traditionally stored in snowbanks until needed in
the kitchen. Many of these dishes come from the regions that also
staff most Indian restaurants in North America. Cookbook author
and curry specialist Camella Panjabi explains that most Indian
restaurateurs—on both continents—are Punjabi, an ethnicity rooted
in the mountains of Northern India and thus reliant on some of the
same greens and root crops familiar to winter gardeners here.

Indian food is typically served not course by course but all at
once, with a sampling of carefully flavored dishes along with lots
of rice and flatbreads to absorb and mix the intriguing tastes.

Broccoli Dal Curry

Watercress Raita

Basmati Rice

Naan

Carrot Halvah

japanese

· ·

There's nothing imaginative about this combination, but that
doesn't make it less tasty.

Miso Soup

Turnip Salad

Tempura

Rice

north african

North African cooking is the lesser-known aspect of the much-touted Mediterranean diet. Like its cousins, it features olive oil, lots of vegetables or pasta and rice. The pasta is generally in the form of couscous rather than noodles. Also, spices tend to be more complex and emphatic, and meat, when served, will be lamb, chicken, or fish, rather than beef or pork.

Moroccan Carrot Salad

Moroccan Squash Purée

Couscous

Swiss Chard and Olives with Preserved Lemons

turkish

Like many long contested areas of the world, Turkey is home to a complex and sophisticated cuisine that deserves a wider audience. Middle Eastern, South Asian, and European traditions combine to memorable pilafs, flaky pastries, stuffed vegetables, and layered casseroles. One winter Anatolian custom is to get together between December 22 and January 30, by tradition the coldest days of winter, and feast on filled savory pastries and halvah. If you decide to add such as evening to your winter social schedule, don't forget to serve mint tea and sweet strong coffee.

Hortopita **(This is officially Greek, but I've had nearly identical treats, called borek, from a street cart in Istanbul)**

Cauliflower and Lentil Stew

Earth Apples in Olive Oil

Pilaf

Salad

a festive vegan meal

Roasted Cauliflower Hidden Garlic Soup

Simmered Fennel

Polenta

Grilled Portabella Mushrooms

Quince Sorbet

gluten-free

Brussels Sprout Salad

Haricot Mélange

Rice

Baked Sweet Potato Snack Strips

Carrot Torte

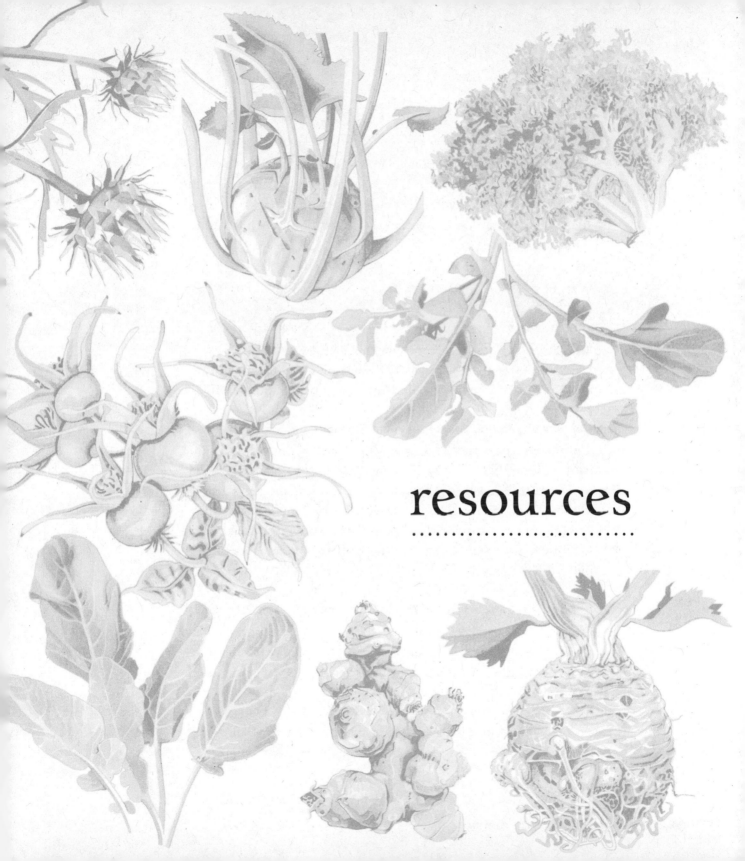

resources

RESOURCES

Finding specific information about winter crops and recipes is not the challenge it used to be. What follows makes no attempt to be inclusive. It is a highly idiosyncratic collection of books, Internet sites, and plant and seed sources that I have found helpful and thought-provoking.

books

I didn't pick winter cookbooks for this list. If you're reading this, you already have one! These are books that have expanded my ideas about food, menus, and eating thoughtfully and happily.

The New Vegetarian Epicure, by Anna Thomas

I learned to cook in college, in group houses with gardens in the back and the *Vegetarian Epicure* and *Tassajara Bread Book* on the shelves. After 20 years, Thomas returned to cookbook writing in the 1990s with her familiar verve, passion for good food, and a lighter, more family-oriented approach to meatless cooking. Reading her recipes is like chatting with an old friend as we make dinner together.

Risotto, by Judith Barrett and Norma Wasserman

I've made at least a dozen of the risotti in this collection, and every one has been terrific. The authors' clear, friendly explanations guide cooks toward their own variations.

A Mediterranean Harvest, by Paola Scaravelli and Jon Cohen

This is where I first learned about North African and Turkish recipes, along with the more familiar Mediterranean cuisines.

Seafood is covered but no other meat, which leaves room for all sorts of intriguing vegetable treatments.

Flatbreads and Flavors: A Baker's Atlas, by Jeffrey Alford and Naomi Duguid

Bread is the heart of most traditional cuisines, and flatbreads are the basis of rural and nomadic cooking on most continents. This book takes some time to sort out, arranged as it is by culture rather than by course, but it is wonderful. The authors' vignettes from their adventurous culinary travels are worth the price.

Crossroads Cooking: The Meetings and Mating of Ethnic Cuisines—from Burma to Texas, by Elisabeth Rozin

Rozin specializes in historic and ethnic cuisine, and this book combines this expertise with over 200 recipes illustrating how the tides of war and commerce have influenced our cooking. Every one I've tried has been terrific.

The Voluptuous Vegan, by Myra Kornfeld with George Minot

I learned a lot from this book. Creating full and balanced flavors without meat or dairy takes skill, and the authors are up to the challenge. Techniques may be multi-step and take some time, so I save most of these recipes for company meals, but they are not difficult, and most can be made without a lot of esoteric ingredients.

The Omnivore's Dilemma, by Michael Pollan

This is hardly a neglected title, but I can't leave it out. Lucid, provocative, and full of respect for real food and what it takes to produce it, it's a magnificent book.

Growing Vegetables West of the Cascades, Steve Solomon

Steve Solomon founded the Territorial Seed Company and was one of the first seed sellers to specialize in cool weather crops. He is erudite and opinionated, and any of the several editions of his gardening books are worth having.

Gardening When It Counts: Growing Food in Hard Times, by Steve Solomon

Like most things that get trendy, the quest for local, seasonal food can quickly lose sight of basic realities. Steve Solomon is great for bringing us back to Earth, both figuratively and literally. If my absolute top concerns were food self-sufficiency and minimal use of resources, I would stop fooling around with my finicky Meyer lemon and the tubs of eggplants on my deck and concentrate on how to produce the most nutrients with the least input of water, fertilizer, and human energy. For those with the room to do it, maybe 1,000 square feet per eater, Solomon advocates quitting the intensive raised-bed methods that have been home gardeners' standard since the 1970s and going back to wider plant spacings, less water, more judicious use of fertilizers, and potatoes, lots of potatoes.

Winter Gardening in the Maritime Northwest, by Binda Colebrook

Long out of print, but available through used booksellers and libraries, this is the classic that I first learned from. Binda has inspired generations of gardeners to get out there and plant that kale. Her advice on soil amendments and fertilizing for cool-weather crops is particularly specific and helpful.

Gardening at the Dragon's Gate, by Wendy Johnson

A one-of-a-kind meditation guide and memoir of gardening and Zen practice.

The Encyclopedia of Country Living, by Carla Emery and her many, many correspondents over 25 years. (Disclosure: I was a fact-checker for the 9th edition, and it contains some recipes from the first Winter Harvest.)

From its first incarnation in 1969 as a set of mimeoed papers in a three-ring binder through to the 10th edition, published posthumously in 2008, this book is a sort of cultural diary of late-20th-century back-to-the-land experiences. Part journal, part encyclopedia, and occasional religious tract, it combines Carla's outsized personality with a staggering range of information. It covers everything from digging wells to giving pills to cows, to growing parsnips. No book so inclusive can cover everything thoroughly, even at 900 pages, but nothing I've read gives the flavor of family homesteading as well as this. Carla lived in Kendrick, Idaho, so much of her experience has a Northwest (though not maritime) flavor.

The Savory Wild Mushroom, by Margaret McKenny

I grew up with this venerable mushroom guide. It was published in 1962, and I've never been without one since. It's easy to use, oriented toward Northwest species, and it contains a classic essay on mushroom foraging by Angelo Pellegrini, a cautionary treatise on mushroom toxins, and a recipe for chanterelle fritters that makes me long for fall to come.

websites and blogs

Gardening with Carol

Carol McIntyre gardens, publishes, and teaches on winter gardening from her home in Merville, BC, north of Comox on Vancouver Island. Her "Full Circle" winter-gardening seminar course has been refined over the past 10 years, and she publishes a teaching calendar for winter growers.

winter-harvestvegetables.ca

Whatcom Locavore

Nancy Ging is an artist and island dweller who blogs about her quests for great food grown or produced in Whatcom County, WA.

whatcomlocavore.com

The Chatelaine's Keys

Sharon Astyk is a book author, prolific blogger, farmer in upstate New York, teacher and mom. She takes on the paradox of resource depletion and personal abundance in a way that makes you think hard, while making pickles. Her energy and erudition fairly vibrate on the screen of her blog — The Chatelaine's Keys — at **sharonastyk.com.**

Northwest Garden History

A labor of love from botanist and historian Kathy Mendelson, this site tracks notable gardeners, gardens, and plant varieties in the Pacific Northwest. It has set me on a quest for the Oregon giant bean, popular in the 1920s and reported to germinate in cold soil and set foot-long pods. **halcyon.com/tmend/plants.htm**

Old Northwest Foodie Thinks It Through

I also have a blog—more active sometimes than others—where I write about local foods and city gardening.
nwlocalfoods.blogspot.com

Slow Food USA

Among many other programs, the Slow Food movement supports heritage vegetable varieties through its Ark of Taste project, conecting gardeners and cooks with suppliers to keep great-tasting endangered vegetable varieties in production. Their choices include the Inchelium red garlic from Eastern Washington, and the Ozette fingerling potato. **slowfoodusa.org**

The Ethicurean: Chew the Right Thing

A wonderful umbrella site for anyone who cares about both taste and the big picture—equity, environment, economics—when it comes to food. **ethicurean.com**

seeds and plants

These Pacific Northwest businesses all provide local expertise and cool weather varieties.

TERRITORIAL SEED COMPANY
PO Box 158
Cottage Grove, OR 97424
Phone Orders: 800-626-0866
Customer Service/Gardening Questions: 541-942-9547
territorialseed.com

Looking through Territorial's history on its website, I realize that I must have been an early customer. Their first catalog was published in late 1979, and I was planting their Northwest-tested seeds by early 1981. One of the many things I have appreciated about Territorial right from the start is that the "days to maturity" estimates are actually calibrated to Northwest summers, which often don't really get going until well into July. I could stop adding three weeks to the estimates given by companies that test their plants in Iowa or North Carolina. Another mark in their favor is that they were the first, and still one of the few, to focus on winter gardening. They have produced a separate winter catalog for more than 20 years.

NICHOLS GARDEN NURSERY
1190 Old Salem Rd NE
Albany, OR 97321
Phone: 800-422-3985
nicholsgardennursery.com

I'll let these long-time Oregon suppliers speak for themselves. "Nichols is proudly celebrating our 60th anniversary in 2010. This is an exciting time at our nursery. In this time of corporate culture and takeovers, we remain a family-operated business, steeped in a tradition of customer service and fine food gardening. We are an original signer of the Safe Seed Pledge and offer no genetically modified seeds or plants. Nichols does not sell or offer treated seed." Many open-pollinated varieties featured.

WILD GARDEN SEED
PO Box 1509
Philomath, OR 97370
Phone: 541-929-4068
wildgardenseed.com

Five varieties of chicory, 16 kinds of mustard, 4 types of orach: you get the idea. This is the place for wild and barely domesticated greens of various types, organically grown in Oregon. They are also working toward salable amounts of heirloom garden vegetables, including open-pollinated Bloomsdale Savoy spinach (my personal favorite) and golden chard. Not a full-service company, unless you don't care to grow tomatoes, peas, beans or summer squash, but great for winter vegetables.

CLOUD MOUNTAIN FARM
6906 Goodwin Rd.
Everson, WA 98247
Phone: 360-966-5859
cloudmountainfarm.com

Tom and Cheryl Thornton have been specializing in locally adapted fruit varieties for more than 20 years and have educated thousands of Northwest Washington gardeners. Their annual Fall Fruit Festival, usually the first weekend in October, is the best chance you'll get to sample new and heirloom varieties of grapes, apples, pears, kiwis, and most any other fruit that can be grown around here. They also will arrange inspections and phytosanitary certificates to clear the way for Canadian customers taking plants back across the border.

RAINTREE NURSERY
391 Butts Rd.
Morton, WA 98356
Phone: 1-800-391-8892
raintreenursery.com

Raintree has been around since 1972 and markets all over the
US, but it is based in the Cascade Foothills near Morton, Washington. It has a huge array of fruit trees, vines and bushes. One
innovation is to sell preserves made from some of its more unusual
varieties—such as Chinese quince, Rossina mountain ash, and
Aronia berries—so that customers can try out the flavors before
committing to the plants.

RONNIGER POTATO FARM LLC
12101 2135 Rd.
Austin, CO 81410
Phone: 877-204-8704
ronnigers.com

Ronniger's got started in northern Idaho in the 1970s and helped
to bring back dozens of specialty potato varieties. If you've had the
chance to fall in love with the flavor of Yellow Finns, you probably
can thank Jim Ronniger. Decades later, the company has moved
out of and back into family ownership and relocated to Colorado.
It sells specialty onions and Jerusalem artichokes as well as a
dizzying variety of spuds, including the sublime Ozette fingerlings, grown by the Makah on the Olympic Peninsula since the
late 18th century.

canadian suppliers

WEST COAST SEEDS
3925 64th St., RR#1
Delta, BC V4K 3N2
Phone: 604-952-8820
westcoastseeds.com

A great resource for information as well as organic open-pollinated seed. Offering seeds and support for short-season and winter gardeners, including a free guide: **westcoastseeds.com/admin/files/west-coast-seeds-winter-guide.pdf**

FULL CIRCLE SEEDS
PO Box 807
Sooke, BC, Canada V9Z 1H8
Phone: 250-642-3671

Organic, untreated, open-pollinated seeds. A great source for a huge variety of salad greens.

STELLAR SEEDS
S6 C5, RR #1
Sorrento, BC V0E 2W0
Phone: 250-675-0076
stellarseeds.com

Sells regionally grown, open-pollinated, organic seeds, and is one of the few places I know to order scorzonera seed. They also offer bulk orders for market growers.

RECIPE INDEX

· ·

V (*vegan*)   **VT** (*vegetarian*)   **GT** (*gluten-free*)

index

about the author

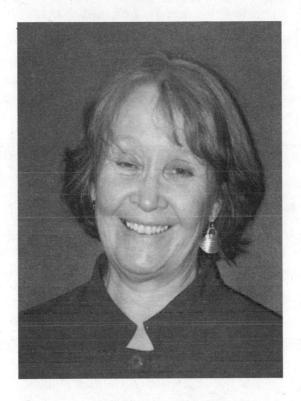

Lane Morgan has written and contributed to several books on food and history, including the *Pacific Northwest the Beautiful Cookbook, The Territorial Seed Company Cookbook, The Good Food Guide to Washington and Oregon, Greetings from Washington, The Miracle Planet*, and the *Northwest Experience anthologies*. She is a recipient of the Washington Governor's Writers Award. She has been a homesteader, college professor, journalist, and editor, and currently teaches high school. She lives in Bellingham, Washington.

If you have enjoyed *Winter Harvest Cookbook*, you might also enjoy other

BOOKS TO BUILD A NEW SOCIETY

Our books provide positive solutions for people who want to
make a difference. We specialize in:

**Sustainable Living • Green Building • Peak Oil
Renewable Energy • Environment & Economy
Natural Building & Appropriate Technology
Progressive Leadership • Resistance and Community
Educational & Parenting Resources**

New Society Publishers

ENVIRONMENTAL BENEFITS STATEMENT

New Society Publishers has chosen to produce this book on recycled paper made
with **100% post consumer waste,** processed chlorine free, and old growth free.

For every 5,000 books printed, New Society saves the following resources:[1]

54	Trees
4,864	Pounds of Solid Waste
5,352	Gallons of Water
6,981	Kilowatt Hours of Electricity
8,843	Pounds of Greenhouse Gases
38	Pounds of HAPs, VOCs, and AOX Combined
13	Cubic Yards of Landfill Space

[1]Environmental benefits are calculated based on research done by the Environmental Defense Fund
and other members of the Paper Task Force who study the environmental impacts of the paper
industry.

For a full list of NSP's titles, please call 1-800-567-6772 *or check out our website* at:

www.newsociety.com

NEW SOCIETY PUBLISHERS
Deep Green for over 30 years